# CHOOSE LIFE

By

**Reverend Monsignor James J. Mulligan**

**The Pope John Center**
186 Forbes Road
Braintree, Massachusetts

*Imprimatur:*

Most Reverend Thomas J. Welsh, J.C.D., D.D.
Bishop of Allentown

Copyright © 1991
by
The Pope John XXIII Medical-Moral
Research & Education Center
Braintree, MA 02184

**Library of Congress Cataloging-in-Publication Data**

Mulligan, James J.
   Choose Life/by James J. Mulligan
   p. 383 cm.
   Includes bibliographical references and index.
   ISBN 0-935372-31-8 : $17.95
   1. Catholic Church. Congregatio pro Doctrina fidei. Donum vitae.
2. Catholic Church — Doctrine. 3. Human reproductive technology —
Religious aspects — Catholic Church. 4. Medical ethics. I. Title.
RG133.5.M85 1991
241'.66—dc20                                  91—31394
                                              CIP

This book is lovingly dedicated to the
memory of my parents,

Edmund and Rose Mulligan,

who, by word and example,
taught me that life is sacred.

# TABLE OF CONTENTS

# FOREWORD

In February of 1987 the Congregation for the Doctrine of the Faith issued its *Instruction on Respect for Human Life in its Origin and on the Dignity of Procreation.* The instruction, like most such documents, was intended to be of practical help to people. Unfortunately, the language of such instructions is, of necessity, technical and sometimes obscure to those for whom it is ultimately intended. This is true in many areas — even in medicine, which is so obviously also intended, in the final analysis, to be of practical help to real people.

In 1989 I began to write a column called "Moral Decisions" for the *A.D. Times,* the diocesan newspaper of the Diocese of Allentown. It has since begun to appear in many other Catholic newspapers as well. I had for many years been a teacher of medical ethics at Mount Saint Mary's Seminary in Emmitsburg, Maryland. In the course of teaching I learned a great deal about the need to make the technical understandable. It became my purpose, therefore, to write a column that would open to its readers, in clear language, the ideas and principles so important to them and yet made so obscure by the sesquipedalian vocabulary of the medical practitioner or the theological *peritus* — and to do so without recourse to the excessively long and overly complex sentences to which one is so often subjected in the literature of those particular areas of expertise. In other words, I wanted to get away from the sort of writing that you just saw in that last sentence.

I also decided to write the first series of columns on that 1987 *Instruction* to which I referred earlier. This book is based on the original columns, but is not by any means a simple reprinting of them. The column format has some severe restraints by reason of the fact that space is so limited. A book allows for more explanation, better continuity and room for reflection. And that is how this present volume comes now to be inflicted on an unsuspecting public.

A foreword is also a place in which to express thanks. This one is no exception. I would like to thank Reverend Robert G. Cofenas and Deacon John J. Murphy, former and present editors of the *A.D. Times*. I must also thank the Most Reverend Thomas J. Welsh, Bishop of Allentown, who has encouraged me in my writing and who has given me an assignment in which it is possible to find time to write. I thank the Most Reverend Joseph McShea, the retired Bishop of Allentown, who assigned me to Mount Saint Mary's Seminary in 1963 and so gave me the chance to pursue my interest in theology.

I thank, too, my former colleagues and students at Mount Saint Mary's Seminary, where I gained my experience in teaching. Foremost among them I should thank the Most Reverend Harry J. Flynn, Bishop of Lafayette in Louisiana, since it was he, as rector of the Seminary, who first got me involved in this particular area of theology.

Finally, I offer sincere thanks to Mrs. Maria A. Loch, a secretary with infinite patience, who typed and retyped columns and manuscript with words of encouragement rather than complaint, and then even undertook the job of doing the typesetting of the book as well.

# CHAPTER 1
## THE POPE IN THE BEDROOM

"The Pope should stay out of the bedroom." You may recall hearing that statement or something similar to it back in 1987, when the Congregation for the Doctrine of the Faith issued an instruction which began with the words, *Donum vitae,* the gift of life. Its title was *Instruction on Respect for Human Life in its Origin and on the Dignity of Procreation.*[1]

"The Pope should stay out of the bedroom." It was one of those clever but empty-headed comments that skirts its way around the truth in an effort to head off serious consideration. It tries to make you laugh before you think. It is, perhaps, on a par with, "Can anything good come from Nazareth?"[2] It gives you permission to smile knowingly and then walk away without ever really looking.

---

[1]Congregation for the Doctrine of the Faith, *Instruction on Respect for Human Life in its Origin and on the Dignity of Procreation,* February 22, 1987, hereafter referred to as *Instruction.* The full text of the instruction (in the translation reprinted by the Pope John Research Center) is contained in an appendix to this book. I have numbered the paragraphs for easier reference, and all footnotes will use those numbers.

[2] Jo 1,46

1

What are the implications of such a statement? It certainly implies that there are some areas of personal life into which the Church, or even religion, should not enter. But, why not? Are those areas too insignificant to bother with? Are they too secular to be touched by religion? Are they too personal? Too intimate?

The *Instruction* deals with questions of biomedical ethics and morality. It considers human life from the moment of its conception. It looks at current concerns in respect to human life within the womb. It takes up the all too frequent and deeply painful problem of infertility. It asks serious questions and proposes significant responses. Surely none of these areas is too insignificant to be of concern to the Church.

There is nothing insignificant about the power to create new human life. Even if it were simply a question of the physical capacity to beget and bear a child, that in itself would be far from insignificant. But begetting and birth are just the beginning. The creation of a human being is a gradual process, starting with nine months of intra-uterine life and continuing through long, and frequently difficult, years of love, nurturance and guidance that finally produce the adult daughter or son of God. It is indeed significant. So significant that the Church *had better* be concerned about it.

The Church has its faults, for its members and its leaders are sinful human beings. Still, it is and remains the Body of Christ. The love of God is not an abstraction, an empty ideal, a lifeless thing. It is a living reality made present to us in real people, in a living community with its real leaders. It is into that community that every new member is born through Baptism.

2

This is why the Church is so concerned about every marriage and about every act in which the power to procreate is present. This is why it pays so much attention to the relationship of husband and wife. This is why, in the very practical realm of life, it tries to take so much interest in the way people prepare for marriage and go about the process of the creation of new life.

The Church, universal and local, tries to establish norms for preparation prior to marriage, even making them part of its rule of life. These are expressions of love and concern. They are intended to bring a woman and man to see and reflect on the seriousness of their love for each other and for God. The Church intends what they also intend and desire — that they may enter into a union that will be as deep and as full as ever a union of frail creatures may be.

It is in this loving union that they will live and grow together. It is into this union that new life will be born. There is hardly anything more significant or more worthy of the Church's fullest attention and concern.

Are there any areas of life which are so completely secular that the Church should refrain from entering into them? There are surely areas in which the Church does not and never has claimed a special competence.[3] It would not, for example, presume to make medical diagnoses, nor would it claim that its competence extended to physics or chemistry or bus schedules or cookery. But in any area it can and should be concerned about the moral dimensions of

---

[3] "The Church's Magisterium does not intervene on the basis of a particular competence in the area of experimental sciences; but having taken account of the data of research and technology, it intends to put forward, by virtue of its evangelical mission and apostolic duty, the moral teaching corresponding to the dignity of the person and to his or her integral vocation." (*Instruction*, n.3).

3

life. It can very well make moral statements about the uses of arsenic in soup or cyanide in Tylenol. It can and should be concerned that the use of chemistry may result in horrifying weapons or dangerous pesticides. Their use has a most significant moral implication. It must take notice of and comment upon the use of physics to improve and promote atomic weaponry. It can, without claiming competence to diagnose the state of one's health, make absolutely necessary statements about what is done in the process of diagnosis or what happens to a human being as a result of diagnosis.

There is no shadow of doubt that the Church is operating fully within its competence when it comments upon methods of procreation and the sacredness of new life. It does not claim authority to diagnose causes of infertility, but it would be shirking a sacred trust if it failed to make any moral judgment on the bewildering variety of possibilities that medicine might propose as solutions.

The secular world is not an entity unto itself merely coexisting, side by side, with the sacred. It is, rather, a world which needs redemption and needs the dimension of the sacred to give it full meaning. Were there no point of union between the two, our lives would be perfect examples of the split personalities which used to be diagnosed as schizophrenic. The effort to live in a purely secular world would give us a plethora of possibilities, always devoid of final meaning. The Church is untrue to itself and untrue to God as well if it stands by in silence and allows that to happen.

"Thanks to the progress of the biological and medical sciences, man has at his disposal ever more effective therapeutic resources; but he can also acquire new powers, with unforeseeable consequences, over human life at its very beginning and in its first stages. Various procedures now make it possible to intervene not only in order to assist but also to dominate the process of procreation. These techniques can enable man to 'take in hand his own destiny,' but they also expose him 'to the temptation to go beyond the limits of a reasonable dominion over nature.' They might constitute progress in the service of man, but they also involve serious risks. Many people are therefore expressing an urgent appeal that in interventions on procreation the value and rights of the human person be safeguarded. Requests for clarification and guidance are coming not only from the faithful but also from those who recognize the Church as 'an expert in humanity' with a mission to serve the 'civilization of love' and of life."[4]

Is the area of procreation so personal and so intimate, that the Church should not enter into it? There should be no doubt at all about its personal and intimate nature. Its intimacy is not only a *fact* of the relationship, it is also a *quality* to be nurtured and deepened. The physical reality of the sexual relationship is a sad and shallow, self-serving and self-seeking act without the depth of intimate, personal, exclusive love. This is precisely the problem and one source of the pain which emerges from promiscuity, fornication and adultery.

For the Christian, sexuality has a dimension that goes far beyond physical or emotional desire. Intercourse is far more than an act in which physical conception can occur. It is an intimate expression of living and life-giving love, a concrete reflection of God's own creative power.

---

[4] *Instruction*, n. 2.

5

The Church is concerned about this reality, *not in spite of* the fact that it is so personal and intimate, but *because* it is so. To say that something is personal and intimate and, therefore, beyond the scope of the Church's concern is to speak nonsense. It is to say that God and Church and religion belong on the fringes and the surface of our existence, but should not penetrate to its depths. It would result in a foolish effort to live while not allowing God to touch or enter into what is most important.

This is why the Church is and *must be* concerned about sexuality and procreation. I have heard the objection voiced that the Church is overly preoccupied with matters sexual. The implication, of course, is that society at large is not. It would seem to me that such an objection would best be made by an ostrich who has spent his whole life with his head in the sand. Look at advertising. Look at the newspapers. Watch almost any program of any sort on television. Go to almost any motion picture. Then come back and tell me that references to sex were minimal and showed no signs of preoccupation. I will be happy to help you find an ophthalmologist and to direct you to someone who can help you with your hearing loss. Or I can help you find your way back to the sandbox.

The world around us is preoccupied with sex, and it frequently has not a clue as to its meaning. When the Church addresses issues of sexuality, it is addressing a need which is pervasive in our society. It may well be that the Church is the only non-ostrich left in the midst of an epidemic of head burying. It is one of the few institutions unafraid to look at the truth and express it. It knows when the Emperor has no clothes. It had better be concerned about the real meaning and value of sex, because precious few others seem to be. Too many want the fun and games of sex, the simple (and hurtful) use of others, without the

6

love and fidelity and responsibility that give it real meaning.

"The gift of life which God the Creator and Father has entrusted to man calls him to appreciate the inestimable value of what he has been given and to take the responsibility for it: this fundamental principle must be placed at the center of one's reflection in order to clarify and resolve the moral problems raised by artificial interventions on life as it originates and on the process of procreation."[5]

Science does have its rightful place in the process of the origin of life. I will look quite carefully at that in later chapters. For the moment, however, it seems enough to say that there is a clear and foolish lack of logic in saying, "Keep the Pope out of the bedroom — but open wide the doors and usher in a host of biologists, doctors and technicians!"

---

[5]*Instruction,* n.1.

# CHAPTER 2

## SEEING THE WHOLE ELEPHANT

There is a fable about a group of blind men who had never been exposed to an elephant. They were introduced to one and then told to describe it. One had touched its trunk and had no doubt that an elephant was much like a snake. Another had touched a leg and was certain that it was far more like a tree trunk. The one who felt its ear knew to a certainty that the others were mistaken — an elephant was similar to a broad-leafed plant. Of course, everyone was right — and everyone was wrong. No one had grasped it all, so no one could put it all together.

The sciences — and here my emphasis would be on biology and medicine — have blossomed in this century. I am sure that I would not be far wrong to say that in the last fifty years they have discovered more than they did in all the years which preceded. Nor has it been a matter of simple accumulation of information. Knowledge has not remained trapped in the ivied halls of academe, but has been put to practical use.

Biochemical discoveries have led to new possibilities for drugs and therapy. One need only look at the more than 2400 large pages of very small print, which make up the 1989 edition of the *Physician's Desk Reference*. One would almost be tempted to think that we must have drugs available for diseases that haven't even been invented yet. Yet, it is at times a bit frightening to find buried in their description the comment that a number of them work, although no one is certain exactly why or how. Or to realize that many of them can or do have quite serious and undesirable side effects. Or that all of their side effects — especially long range, genetic ones — have not yet been available for study.

Mechanical and electronic inventions have led to medical techniques hardly envisioned just a few years ago. Ways of imaging internal organs or looking deeply enough to see the inner structure and functions of single cells have opened up vast realms of heretofore impossible interventions. Transplants, not only of living organs but even of mechanical devices, have brought us into a world that a few decades back would have been the exclusive province of science fiction.

Increased knowledge inevitably has the capacity to bring increased benefits to humanity — and, just as inevitably, it has the potential for increased risks. Increased knowledge also leads to increased specialization. One of the side effects of that is a sort of tunnel vision. It becomes harder for any one person to know a great deal about everything, so there is a tendency, instead, for each to try to learn all there is to be learned about one's own area of expertise. (This, of course, lends some credence to the person who defined the specialist as one who learns more and more about less and less, until at last, he knows everything about nothing). Knowledge deepens, while the field of vision becomes constantly narrower. Perhaps nowhere is this more true than in the study of the process of procreation.

There was a time in the not too distant past when problems of infertility were a matter of puzzlement, frustration and the source of a great deal of self-reproach. Knowledge brought further hope. The functioning of the ovaries and testes could be examined. It became possible to find out if the complicated duct systems of both male and female were capable of properly performing their tasks. Better understanding brought with it greater potential for intervention and assistance.

There are now possibilities of intervention at the levels of micro-surgery, reproductive endocrinology, *in vitro* and *in vivo* fertilization, intra-fallopian transfers, and numberless varieties of other techniques. Within such a host of possibilities, there is a constantly increasing need for specialization, and so a constant narrowing of scope. This can create problems, but at the same time we should not become blind to the fact that this growing body of knowledge has enormous potential to serve the good of humanity — not only humanity in the abstract, but real men and women.

The role of the Church is essential. It is not the Church's function to make judgments on the scientific *facts* which may emerge from such study. It is, however, the Church's function to examine the *moral values* which must be taken into account in the application of those facts to human life — and even to the methods and means by which such facts are uncovered. The Church would be remiss in its duty if it were to ignore this area.

While the Church is quite willing to recognize both its duty and the limits of its scope, this is not always equally true of science. There are all too many who trumpet the advance of science, but have a woefully inadequate grasp of the wider vision of moral concerns. This, of course, is the risk of the necessarily narrowing view of the specialist. He must broaden his focus once in a while, and look out at the rest of the world and the implications of his own area of expertise.

The cytologist, who studies the structure and function of cells, would be clearly and sadly mistaken if he were to try to define the human person as nothing more than a conglomeration of cells. The biologist would be in error if he saw the individual human being as no more than a collection of interrelated, functioning organs. The fertility expert would be equally wrong to see human procreation as no more than a joining of cells without reference to the beginning of a new *person*. The fact is that every area of the study of human life becomes not only narrow, but even absolutely misleading, when it is seen in isolation and loses the relationship it should have to the vision of human life as the life of knowing, loving and interrelated persons. It begins, indeed, to dehumanize as soon as it loses the awareness of human beings as related to God.

The Church's function is, at times, to remind science that it can assist in procreation, but must not dominate it. It must never think that it is dealing with cells to be manipulated, when it is actually dealing with persons to be loved and respected. It is the job — the sacred duty — of the Church to call attention to the criteria of moral judgement. "These criteria are the respect, defence and promotion of man, his primary and fundamental right to life, his dignity as a person who is endowed with a spiritual soul and with moral responsibility and who is called to beatific communion with God."[6]

The moral teaching of the Church does not come simply from a sense of "duty," nor even from a need to carry out some sort of "function." It emerges, instead, from a real

---

[6] *Instruction*, n. 3.

care and concern and love for persons.[7]  Its purpose is to
open their minds and their hearts.  A grasp of morality
brings with it a widening of vision.  When we see ourselves
and others as children of God, demanding love and respect
and dignity, then our point of view on everything else
becomes what it ought to be.

The Church's moral teaching is not and never has been,
a mere set of rules.  It is not designed simply to command,
but to instruct.  It does not decide for us what we are to do;
rather, it gives us the information and insight that enable us
to know *what* we are to do and *why*.  It sets us free of the
domination of a partial knowledge that could mislead and
even destroy.  It shows us what we are and who we are, so
that we can act with the greatest respect for ourselves and
for others.  It gives meaning to what could otherwise be
seen as no more than mechanical acts — and it shows us
when our actions are such that they undermine and begin to
destroy what we really are.

A moral theology which took no account of scientific fact
would be as inadequate as a science which had no grasp of
moral theology.  The Church, in its teaching and documents, tries to add depth to our awareness of ourselves by
bringing together the best elements of both.  How sad it is
that so often our grasp of science and morality comes to us
through the filter of news media, which know hardly
anything about either.  We owe it to ourselves to learn far
more.

We are all tempted at times to judge all of reality on the
basis of quite limited views, needs and desires.  The
teaching of the Church constantly calls us back to a wider

---

[7] Cf. *Instruction*, nn. 4-5.

vision of the dignity, value and worth of each human being at every moment of life. What a sad thing it would be if we never took the time to look at the whole elephant!

# CHAPTER 3
## IN SEARCH OF SUPER RAT

At the risk of sounding like a commentary on *60 Minutes*, I have a question for you. Have you ever noticed that hardly a week goes by without at least one news release on a product that was removed from the market because it had been found to cause cancer in rats? Does it ever make you wonder who is in charge?

I recall reading an article some years ago in which the author suggested that in laboratories it is really the rats who are in charge and they are gradually getting rid of anything that can be harmful to them.[8] Will the day finally come when we are all dead and gone, and the world will be ruled by the healthiest rats it has ever known?

That fear is, perhaps, unfounded. But the frequency of the reports do point out how common it is for products to be developed and rushed to market, and only then be revealed to have flaws which may be not only dangerous but deadly.

The speed with which new discoveries are made available for use is certainly indicative of the sorts of problems that science can face as it forges rapidly ahead without full awareness of the results of its own actions. Such rapidity

---

[8] Alas, I cannot recall the source of this story, but it may well have been in *The Journal of Irreproducible Results*.

is due, to some extent, to the expected enthusiasm of scientists anxious to let their work be known. It is more often, I would suspect, due to the prospect of commercial gain by the scientists themselves or the companies who hire them. Pressures for profit lead to cutting corners on testing and so to serious harm. They also lead to promotion of drugs or techniques without due consideration for their moral implications. Damage is bad enough when it is physical; it is far worse when it is moral. The combination of science and commerce is, I suppose, unavoidable. Yet neither science nor commerce are *in themselves* adequate judges of morality.

The Book of Genesis begins with its account of creation, and in it humanity is given dominion over everything on earth.[9] That dominion is certainly to be found in the human capacity for scientific research and its application to human life.[10] Science has enormous potential for good. It must be pointed out, however, that its function is such that it is able to discover what we *can* do. Unfortunately, science, all by itself, tells us nothing at all about what we *should* do. "Science and technology are valuable resources for man when placed at his service and when they promote his integral development for the benefit of all; but they cannot of themselves show the meaning of existence and of human progress."[11]

---

[9] Gen 1,28.

[10] 3. Cf. *Instruction*, n.6.

[11] *Instruction*, n.6.

15

The concept of a "science" was at one time applied to every body of knowledge, including philosophy and theology. At present, however, it is used in a more restricted sense to refer rather exclusively to empirical or experimental bodies of learning. For this reason, our own society often draws a rather clear line between "science" on the one hand, and "theology" on the other. There is also a sadly mistaken tendency to consider the conclusions of science as proven facts, and the conclusions of theology as theory open to simple acceptance or rejection on the basis of personal inclination.

The truth of the matter is that experimental science is simply incapable of certain things. It has some serious limits on what it can do. It can measure bodies, but it cannot weigh the soul. It can look at the physical structure of a cell, but it cannot put good or evil under a microscope. Yet good and evil are certainly more significant in life than is the structure of the cell. The immortal soul is what gives meaning to the body which can be so easily examined.

The fact is that even empirical science is constantly forced into its own "act of faith" because of its own limits. The whole concept of atomic and subatomic particles is taken for granted; but no one has ever seen them. They make perfect sense and the theories which take them into account certainly seem to work in the practical order. But science still cannot see them, because it lacks the tools to do so. Shall we deny their existence because science cannot see them, even though they are within its own area of study? I should think not, for their effects are all too evident. Shall we deny the world of good or evil or morality because science cannot "see" them. I should think not. Their effects are also all too evident. If science has such trouble dealing with its own domain, we should

16

certainly not be at all surprised when it cannot deal with something so far beyond its limits.

We must keep in mind, however, that the results of scientific research are not morally neutral. The application of chemistry to the production of nerve gas has a moral dimension. The use of nuclear physics to produce more terrifying weaponry is not without moral significance. The purpose of science — as, indeed, the purpose of whatever is worthwhile in life — should be the *good* of humanity. Science is itself a tool for our use in the accomplishment of our real goals, and those goals cannot be understood independently of our relationship to God and to each other. The purposes of the sciences are not understood at all when they are seen apart from the person and moral values. This gives science its real meaning and also sets it certain limits.[12] Science, without the guidance of morality, is like a one-legged blind man carrying nitroglycerine across a crowded ice-skating rink. In other words, I would not find its results predictable, and would most likely find them highly undesirable.

A science which loses sight of morality may easily find itself satisfied to focus on its own technical efficiency. This in itself may be taken as sufficient justification for some rather dreadful results. So, apparently, thought the Nazis, who put such skill and effort into the building of more efficient crematoria. They were proud of the fact that Zyklon-B was such a vast improvement over carbon monoxide as an efficient way of murder. That, of course, is an example from the past. We would never act that way today, would we? Still, we do read of anesthetists in the

---

[12]Cf. *Instruction*, n.7.

17

Netherlands who formulate more potent mixtures for efficient euthanasia. Right here at home we are from time to time reminded to take pride in the fact that the lucrative business of murdering the unborn can now be carried on so efficiently and under such sanitary conditions.

Beyond the mere fact of technical efficiency, there is the further aspect of utility. It does not take long, however, to discover that even the apparent usefulness of certain scientific advances does not guarantee their moral desirability. That is especially true when things become commercialized and the needs (or, sometimes, just the desires) of the few are served at the expense of the many. Preservatives and pesticides, for example, have been used by food producers, even though they killed off some of the consumers. Certainly that can happen as a dreadful accident due to honest mistakes; but we have seen other cases as well. Manufacturers and users have fought to keep unsafe products on the market, for fear of loss of profit or payment of damages for liability.

Even popular ideologies have served as a source of moral justification for "scientific" advances which were dreadful in their application. A perfect example is to be found in the racial ideology of the Nazis. They placed the Aryans at the pinnacle of humanity, with all others beneath them. This led to horrors beyond belief. The crippled, the infirm and the retarded became fit subjects for removal from society. All Jews were classified as sub-human and became a population suitable for oppression, experimentation and, finally, extermination. We look back and attempt to convince ourselves that it could never happen now. Yet in our own culture there is a vague "meaningful quality of life" ideology, which holds that life is human only in the full consciousness of unblemished vitality outside the womb. This creates the willingness to view the unborn as

18

a sub-human storehouse of marketable tissue, to treat the handicapped as expendable and to neglect the ill and the elderly — even to the point of not only allowing death but even causing it.

Technical efficiency, utilitarianism and popular ideologies all fail as sources of moral guidance. What they all lack is real respect for persons. Progress and profit become the norm, not love of neighbor. This can be dehumanizing to its victims. It is even more surely dehumanizing to its perpetrators. *The victims are subjected* to an effort to ignore or crush their humanity. They need not yield. The *perpetrators freely choose* to be less than human in their actions. When the Nazis fell they left an almost inconceivable number of dead behind them; but it was the Nazis themselves who had abdicated their humanity, while so many of their victims emerged with greater dignity.

Only an unconditional respect for the value, the rights and the good of each person can lay the real foundation for the moral use of our ever advancing knowledge and technology. This is what faith has to offer and what the Church teaches. Science — left without moral guidance — will never come to this conclusion. Science must have conscience as well as knowledge, for without conscience it leads to ruin.

We must love our neighbor as we love ourselves; and we can never be satisfied with the dubious consolation that we have at least treated others as well as we treat rats.

# CHAPTER 4
## THE BEAT OF THE TOM-TOM

There was a time when the best medical treatment available came with music — and I don't mean the soothing sounds in the waiting room of your dentist. In the good old days the practitioner was a witch doctor in a mask, and he treated his patients with tortoise shell rattles, the beat of a tom-tom and a dance. The theory, of course, made a good deal of sense; otherwise it would never have been so popular. If diseases were caused by evil spirits, then the power of magic might be the best way to drive them out.

There were drawbacks. The theory did not include anatomy, physiology or any concept of how foreign organisms could invade the human body. When I underwent surgery a few years ago, they were still using the masks, but there were no tom-toms, no rattles and not a trace of choreography. Nonetheless, I had great confidence in what they proposed to do; and it seems to have worked, since I am here to tell the tale.

What was the problem with the earlier theory? Well, for one thing, it was completely one-sided. It saw everything in terms of soul or spirit, with little knowledge of the body. Everything was reduced to a matter of malignant spirits or questions of moral good and evil. Its practice may have offered a good bit of consolation to the sufferer, but it was not as helpful as it should have been to the whole person.

20

It is possible today — perhaps it is almost inevitable — that we might fall into another sort of one-sided view. We have gained considerable knowledge of anatomy and physiology. We are able to look even at a patient's internal organs — not only with surgery, but with a whole array of non-invasive techniques. We are quite clear about the origin of a great many diseases — although not, perhaps, so many as one might sometimes think. We have learned how to look into the structure of the cell itself and this has increased our capacity to intervene in most astounding ways in the origin of human life. Lack of knowledge of the body is not our major problem. We have even grown used to the idea that modern medicine can do routinely many things that only a few decades ago might have been considered miraculous.

If we fall into the trap of seeing medicine as a means of manipulating the mechanics and structures of the body, then we too will have a completely one-sided view. In that case modern medicine could, like witchery, become a false consolation. In fact, the trap might be more insidious for us than it was for the witch doctor. He, at least, was aware that there was a dimension beyond his power to manipulate. His methods were occult even to him. Ours are so much more rational that it is easier for us to think that the whole matter is within the dominion of our techniques. That leads us quite readily into a point of view that becomes wholly pragmatic. We can end up dealing totally with bodies, so that medicine becomes mechanics. That possibility is, perhaps, more frightening than the view which sees only spirit. The spiritual view retains a sense that some things are right and others are wrong. The mechanical view looks only at what works and what doesn't.

"Which moral criteria must be applied in order to clarify the problems posed today in the field of biomedicine? The

21

answer to this question presupposes a proper idea of the nature of the human person in his bodily dimension."[13] If our vision of the human person is limited to this life and this world alone, then we are as narrow and one-sided as any witch doctor could ever have been. If our concept of human life focuses on happiness here and now in a material world, and here alone, then we will have no moral norms to speak of, apart from the simple fact that a thing works or does not work within that limited frame of reference.

We must see the *whole* human person, if we want to see medicine and medical practice in the proper light. We must look at the *nature* of humanity in order to have real moral norms. To ask about the nature of a thing is really a very simple question, although we frequently think of it as deeply philosophical. All we are really asking is, "What is this?" Asking that in reference to a human being leads us to the realization that we are *both* body and spirit.

Our moral norms must attend to both body and spirit. Otherwise they will be deceptive and will never touch the whole person. We cannot focus on just one or the other. If we did, it might be quite similar to a person who looked at water and saw that it was composed of oxygen and hydrogen. If he tried to then describe water, not in terms of its totality, but in terms of its parts seen as separate, he would be severely misled. Oxygen supports combustion. Hydrogen is highly explosive. But we do not even pause before we throw water on a fire to extinguish it. The whole thing is, indeed, something more than the sum of its parts.

Body and soul in a human being are not just isolated parts, each seen only in itself and without reference to the

---

[13] Instruction, n.9.

whole person.[14]   Just as the nature of water would never be understood by looking at oxygen and hydrogen separately, so the nature of the human being is not understood by the witch doctor (who sees only spirit) nor by the medical mechanic (who sees only bodily parts).   The body is not just a bundle of tissues, organs and functions.   Not even the body of an animal can be properly understood in that way, if never seen in its living totality.   In the human being, the body can be properly understood only when it is seen as that visible component which, with the soul, constitutes the person who manifests and expresses himself through it. The body is not simply something that a person "possesses," or can simply dispose of as he sees fit.   The body is the person present in this world.   What is done to or by the body is done to or by the person.

True moral norms take all of this into account, and those norms become quite significant in the area of medical practice.   This is especially so since medicine, by its very nature, focuses so fully on the body and therefore runs the risk of dealing with it exclusively.   This also means that moral norms in this area should never be viewed simply as a set of rules which govern action at a kind of biological level.   Instead, those norms are the result of the application of our intelligence to the reality of what we are as full human beings.   We see our bodies as the visible component of a person called to respond in love to God and neighbor. We see them as the visible component of a child of God, a child who deserves to be treated with dignity and respect.

It is, in fact, the loss of that sense of the sacredness of life which, I suspect, has made it possible for doctors now

---

[14] cf. *Instruction*, n.10.

23

to act as abortionists, mercy killers and even public executioners. Once a body is seen only as interrelated working parts, with no concept of soul, it becomes increasingly easier to bring oneself to "dispose" of it.

Over the years I have dealt with many doctors, not only as a patient but in questions of ethics and as a member of hospital ethics committees, and in the vast majority of instances I have been edified by their real care for the whole person. However, there can be in medicine the temptation to deal with patients on some occasions at the level of tissues, organs and functions — forgetting the reality of the fact that persons are spiritual as well. Present attitudes in society make it likely that we shall see in the future an increased number of physicians with this one-sided, mechanistic point of view. This is one reason why it is necessary to promote good laws about determination of death, fetal experimentation and experimental operations or procedures. This is also why there must be clear and serious legislation about the widespread murder of the unborn.

What is lost to sight by some is the moral dimension of medicine. "An intervention on the human body affects not only the tissues, the organs and their functions but also involves the person himself on different levels."[15] There is *always* a moral dimension to be considered when you are working with persons. Medicine works best for the person when it looks at the total, integral good of human life.

"Applied biology and medicine work together for the integral good of human life when they come to the aid of a person stricken by illness and infirmity and when they

---

[15] *Instruction*, n. 12.

24

respect his or her dignity as a creature of God."[16]  Of
course, it is not the function of either medicine or biology,
as science, to be able to determine the origin and destiny of
the human being as person.  The doctor or the biologist
must act in accord with that origin and that destiny, but
does not acquire an awareness of them through medicine or
biology as such.  That knowledge comes from other sources
and then plays a part in the context of the practice of
medicine.  In other words, just as the patient is treated as
a whole and integral person, so also the physician must act
as a whole and integral person.

All that I have been saying applies in a crucial and
critical way in the area of human sexuality and procreation.
There medicine comes into contact with some of bodily
life's most sacred aspects.  The most fundamental values of
love and life are made real and concrete in the relationship
of marriage.[17]  In this area medicine intervenes in a relationship that is "most sacred and most serious,"[18] and
within which occurs the inception of new life.  This
intervention may be helpful.  If it is moral, then it is helpful
to the whole person. On the other hand, if it acts only in
terms of tissue and manipulation and mechanics, then it
becomes immoral and is every bit as one-sided as is the
practice of the witch doctor.

Once again, I emphasize that this is an area in which the
Church *must* speak.  While medicine can and should look

---

[16] *Instruction*, n.13.

[17] Cf. *Instruction*, n. 13.

[18] Words from the *Exhortation* in the old rite of marriage.

to its ability to help people, the Church can and should speak of the meaning of life and from this derive the limits to which we are free to intervene. What is technically possible is not always morally admissible. The tom-tom is certainly not a cure for the whole person. Neither is the drum-roll which heralds every new discovery in medicine.

# CHAPTER 5

## AMOEBAS DON'T DATE

Do you recall your days in high school biology, when you got to peer through a microscope at an amoeba? It squished its way around its little world and as it came across morsels of microscopic matter, it surrounded and digested them. It was busily ingesting nutrients. Well, don't we all? Our manners are better. We use knife and fork and napkin. Our portions are usually more than microscopic. We cook and season and we hardly ever eat anything on the hoof. But we do ingest nutrients. Living things, from the smallest to the largest, need to take in nourishment.

C.S. Lewis, the noted English author, once wrote a sermon entitled, "Transposition."[19] By transposition he was referring to a phenomenon with which we are all actually familiar. It is the way in which things are found at a lower and a higher level, in such a way that they are different at each level and yet are somehow the same. Nutrition is a good example. It is certainly different in the amoeba and the human being, and yet it is somehow the same thing. Allow me to illustrate.

---

[19] C.S. Lewis, "Transposition," in *The Weight of Glory*, Wm. B. Erdmans Publishing Co., Grand Rapids, 1966.

As I said above, the amoeba simply surrounds its food and digests it. Do you have a houseplant? If so, you give it water and, perhaps, even a bit of fertilizer or some plant food. It does not move around and take in particles the way the amoeba does. It is, in fact, much more complex in its digestive system. Water and nutrients are taken in through the roots. Carbon dioxide is "breathed" in through the leaves. Using light and a process called photosynthesis it uses its nourishment to live and grow. There are also, of course, things that it can't do. When you bring it food, does it clap its little leaves and wag its stem? Or does it just sit there, sop up what you put in its pot, and flourish?

Try the same thing with a dog or cat. You'll see a reaction as soon as you break out the food. The cat may be more subtle and give you a few sidelong glances to make sure you're on course as you head for the bowl. The dog may consider the subtle approach a foolish waste of time, jumping around your legs and yapping as he encourages you to get on with it. Get that bowl filled, however, and both cat and dog will look, sniff and either taste or look at you as though you had played a cruel joke and then stalk off or stare and make you feel guilty. They are clearly ready to ingest nutrients, just as an amoeba or a plant would do. But they have given this ingestion business a whole new slant. Their digestive system is more complex, of course, but they have other qualities as well. They are capable of obvious anticipation and they also have preferences. There we have it — the same old need for nutrition which has certainly become at the same time something different than it was in the plant.

And people? Of course we ingest nutrients. We are able to anticipate the pleasure of eating. We have preferences. But we add a dimension no dog or cat has ever been capable of. When a young man calls his favorite girl and asks her to go out on Saturday evening to ingest some nutrients, he is talking about much more than a need for nutrition. The meaning of a meal together is much more than flavor and ingestion. It is not just an invitation to the common trough. There is now a personal dimension far surpassing whatever was taking place in plants or animals. The human meaning of taking someone to dinner is symbolic of a whole range of feelings. It's still nutrition, but it's also something else, a whole new reality at the same time.

Then there is the Eucharist. On the surface isn't it the same old act of ingesting nutrients? And it is infinitely more besides. The eyes see the old, familiar act of eating. Faith sees living union with its Savior. How much the same, and yet how totally different!

What then of reproduction? The single-celled amoeba just splits in half. It reaches a critical size and then divides into two. Amoebas don't date. They don't mate. They don't even have a grasp of basic math. When they want to multiply they divide.

Pollination and seed production in plants are far more complex, but even plants that pollinate each other exhibit no signs of mutual attraction. We may tiptoe through the tulips, but they don't tiptoe to each other. Scientists do not study the courtship rites of carrots, or the mating rituals of begonias. To be sure, the reproductive process of plants is of a much higher order than that of the amoeba, while still being reproduction. In summary: Mating, but no dating.

Then there are animals. Some show signs of attraction. There is the instinctive sexual attraction, sometimes only during very specific mating seasons. It is not the free choice of love, but there may be a form of pair bonding which can be so strong as to keep pairs of some species together for life — a well known example of this is the Canada goose. Animals add a dimension to the reproductive process which makes it exactly what the plants are doing and yet it is at the same time a quite different sort of reality.

Human reproduction is the same reality found in animals, yet it is immensely more. There is, of course, quite an interesting possibility here. Humans have an amazing capacity to become *less* than fully human when they choose to. They can turn sex into an uncaring coupling which results in conception. That might even take them to a level *below* some animals. They can distort their reproductive instinct into mutual use — or abuse — with no idea either of reproduction or care and concern. This ignores even the pair bonding that a goose is capable of. In all of these instances something truly human and humanizing is being lost or even purposely pushed aside. How sad.

Real *human* reproduction is so much more than simple, instinctive pair bonding. The human procreation of life — if it is really and fully human — demands not only fertilization but full and complete personal commitment and marriage is the place where this occurs.

The natural act of eating is for humanity capable of being something more than an animal could ever accomplish. So too is the begetting of a new human life infinitely beyond the possibilities of mere animal reproduction. The Eucharist is far past the level of the usual human partaking of a meal. In the same way Christian sacramental marriage surpasses even the highest level of natural married love. It brings to fully human reproduction the capacity to join in a union bound up in Christ himself and giving rise to new Christian life as a gift to be cherished far beyond mere preservation of the species.

30

"God, who is love and life, has inscribed in man and woman the vocation to share in a special way in his mystery of personal communion and in his work as Creator and Father. For this reason marriage possesses specific goods and values in its union and in procreation which cannot be likened to those existing in lower forms of life. Such values and meanings are of the personal order and determine from the moral point of view the meaning and limits of artificial interventions on procreation and on the origin of human life. These interventions are not to be rejected on the grounds that they are artificial. As such, they bear witness to the possibilities of the art of medicine. But they must be given a moral evaluation in reference to the dignity of the human person, who is called to realize his vocation from God to the gift of love and the gift of life."[20]

Things which may be properly performed in experiments with animals may teach us a great deal about what can be done for human beings. This does not mean, however, that the same things can be done to human beings, nor does it mean that they can always be done in the same way. Experimental procedures in animal fertility, for example, may result in the loss of animal life in its earliest stages. The same procedure in human fertility would result in the loss of the life of a human *person*. That, of course, is quite another matter. The inception of human life should take place in a context of love — a love which finds concrete expression in a bodily act of love. That context does not exist when sperm and ovum are merely collected and then subjected to a technological process which brings about

---

[20] *Instruction*, n. 14.

fertilization in a petri dish.  All of these points, of course, will be examined in more detail in further chapters.

For the moment it is enough to say that the progress of medicine has much to offer in the area of procreation, but the medical practitioner must never lose sight of the fact that he is dealing with *human* life. Full *human* values are to be the guide.  Indeed, the final guide should be full *Christian* values — and that means full respect of each individual human life from the moment of conception.  In us, the power to give life is sacred and is never separate from God and Church.  We are not amoebas.  We are sons and daughters of God.

# CHAPTER 6

## THE STORK: AN ENDANGERED SPECIES?

"Mommy, where do babies come from?" the child asks. "The stork brings them," is the scientific reply. There was a day in which home birth was the norm, and then another favorite answer was, "The doctor brings them in his little black bag." Of course, the stork, like so many birds, moves on and tends eventually to migrate from the land of reality to that of myth. That little black bag, perhaps, does not so easily leave the scene.

Medical intervention in the area of conception increases each year, and within the last twenty years its possibilities have grown more than most of us could ever have imagined. The vocabulary has expanded as fast as have the possibilities. Amniocentesis, sonography and laparoscopy present a range of choices for observation and diagnosis practically from the moment of conception. In fact, intervention can precede conception. We must consider artificial insemination, gamete intrafallopian transfer, removal of tubal occlusion, *in vitro* fertilization, ovarian stimulation and a host of other techniques that are discussed not only in laboratories but in the news media on an almost daily basis. They come up not only as real or potential forms of medical intervention, but also as the source or center of prolonged and painful legal contests. Later we will look at all of those procedures and even more.

In *every* procedure there are moral norms to be considered, since in every one of them we are dealing with the lives of human beings to whom we have moral obligations. That we must never forget. Sounds tiresome, doesn't it? At least there are those who seem to have that impression. They see moral norms as a lot of rules which bore them. Of course, they care about people — that's not only important, it's even rather fashionable. But can't the Church just stop talking about our obligations for a while? I'll decide what's best for me. If you believe that, then you might as well go on believing in the stork, too. You are already living in the world of illusion.

Caring about others is nothing but a mind game if we think that it carries with it no obligations. The day I think that I alone will decide what is right for *me* is the day on which I have lost sight of others. It is when any real caring comes to an end. To know my obligations toward others is really to know how to express any real care or concern for them. That is when I really begin to take them seriously as persons and realize that the result of that care is knowing what I can do or what I ought to do or what I ought not to do. That is when I stop paying lip service to love and really begin loving.

In most areas of life that process of really caring and loving begins with some very basic principles. In the area of procreation the basic concepts are easy enough. "The fundamental values connected with the techniques of artificial human procreation are two: the life of the human being called into existence and the special nature of the transmission of human life in Marriage."[21]

---

[21] *Instruction*, n. 15.

34

The first value is simply that of life itself. It could hardly be more simple or more basic. If I have any real love at all for others, then I should at the very least value their lives. If I do not value the life of the human being who is called into existence by an act of procreation, then I have not even begun to understand the meaning of sex or love or marriage. This is a most fundamental basis for what the Church says about methods of procreation.

*Physical* life in itself does not contain the totality of a person's value. We are called to more than that, since we are called to be and to live as children of God. We are called not only to physical life, but to eternal life. But physical life is fundamental. Upon it all the other values and possibilities of human life are based and developed. No one of us has the right to snuff out another's life for our own gain or convenience or satisfaction.[22]

It is hard ever to justify the taking of anyone's life, even the life of a criminal. It is impossible to justify the direct taking of the life of an innocent person. It does full violence to reason to attempt to justify the creating of innocent life in order to decide to keep a few and snuff out the rest.

The Church is not opposed to techniques of procreation merely on the ground that they are "artificial."[23] It is dead set against those which violate the basic right to life. This is *one* of the problems, for example, with *in vitro* fertilization. The normal procedure for this is to use drugs to stimulate the ovaries. Ordinarily only one egg is produced

---

[22] Cf. *Instruction*, n.16.

[23] Cf. *Instruction*, n.14.

each month.  Stimulation produces many more.  A minimum of seven, usually, are taken from the ovaries and placed in a petri dish where they are fertilized with sperm. They begin to grow —- *each one now a new human being.* Some are placed in the uterus, while the rest are frozen or used for experiment or simply thrown away.

In some instances six or seven are placed in the uterus, with the hope that a few will implant.  If all of them do so, then they cannot all possibly live and come to maturity. Doctors will perform what they like to call "selective reduction."  (We love sanitary terms for dirty procedures.) In plain English, this means, "You have too many children in your uterus.  I am going to kill some of them."

People feeling all the pain of not being able to have children are led step by step on a path which may *possibly produce life,* but will *certainly produce death.*   That is surely a violation of the basic good of life.   Are you surprised that the Church is opposed to it?  Or would you not actually be shocked if the Church did not speak out against it?

The second value has to do with the special nature of the transmission of human life in marriage.  We have already looked at the special quality of human reproduction in the last chapter.  It differs clearly from animal reproduction, because it involves the union of *persons.*   Our sexual activity is not just a blind, animal instinct.  It has become far more than that because we are able to know and love and choose.  Human sexuality is personal and conscious. It is interpersonal and, therefore, its use carries with it obligations — obligations which ought to rise from love.[24]

---

[24] Cf. *Instruction*, n.17.

As a result, we cannot be content with any and every means or method of procreation which happens to work in animals.

There are, indeed, procedures which violate the special nature of the begetting of human life in marriage. The bond of marriage is permanent and exclusive. Artificial insemination with the sperm of a donor (someone other than the husband) is a violation of that fidelity. So also is the use of a husband's sperm to impregnate someone other than his wife — as in "surrogate motherhood." (Please note, once again, how we like to use "artificial insemination by donor" and "surrogate motherhood" as sanitary terms to replace uglier words, such as "infidelity" or "adultery.")

In both of these instances there is clearly no union of husband and wife. In both, sex is reduced to the mechanics of biological reproduction and has lost its character of an intimate expression of personal love between husband and wife. What is also sad and pitiable is the fact that in both instances there is certainly the hope that the real father or real mother will never again be in contact with their children. It really is a dreadful reduction of human sex to mere animal reproduction.

When we purposely destroy the reproductive capability of sex, we do violence to a sacred reality. Taking away the life-giving potential of sex creates a more frightening potential of turning sex into a way of using others for our own pleasure. It is one more violation of the obligation that comes from love.

We do just as much violence to sex when we destroy its intimate and personal dimensions, and reduce it to mere reproduction. The Church teaches that we must preserve both. It presents us with "obligations." But, if we truly love, then we embrace those obligations. When we fail to do so, then we not only violate a "rule" but we begin to tear down relationships and undermine our own humanity. What is morally good builds us up; what is morally wrong begins to unravel the fabric of our lives.

There is much that medicine can and should do. There is also much that it can but should *not* do. "What is technically possible is not for that very reason morally admissible."[25] We have an obligation to know which is which — and that obligation exists because we are called to love each other. From love comes the need to reflect, to think clearly and honestly about those basic values of life and human procreation. Technology which violates those values also violates real persons. The Church merely calls us not to do that.

---

[25] *Instruction*, n.18.

# CHAPTER 7
## TURNING A BLIND EYE

It was the dawn of the Nineteenth Century and Napoleon was out to conquer Europe. It was the day of sail, when silent breezes propelled the stately fleets of tall ships into the thunder of battle. Horatio Nelson — a hero who had lost not only an arm but an eye as well in the service of his country — was sent a signal from the flagship to disengage and break off his attack. He told the signalman on his own ship that he would confirm that order. He took the telescope, held it to his blind eye, and looked through the smoke at the signal flags of the admiral. "I see no such signal," he said. He advanced. He prevailed. He won the day. He faced no court martial. Instead, he was decorated, promoted and went on to even greater fame.

This, perhaps, is the "exception which proves the rule" (whatever that means). In the ordinary course of events, turning a blind eye does not have such happy results. We are almost always better off with both eyes open, knowing where we are headed and how to get there. Not only should our eyes be open, but we should take care that we are not trying to see in the dark. Reason sheds its light on problems, but there is also the light of revelation to be taken into account. What the Church has to say about our humanity, in the light of revelation, opens up more complete and much deeper insight into all that must be known if we are to make the proper decisions in regard to procreation.[26]

The old catechisms used to have a rather matter of fact way of presenting the truths of our faith. They asked clear and simple questions, to which they offered clear and simple answers. One such question was, "Why did God make us?" The answer was, "God made us to know Him, to love Him and to serve Him in the world, and to be happy with Him forever in the next world."

That simple answer has considerable depth of meaning. It tells us, first of all, that we need to know God if we expect even to know ourselves. Knowing God does not mean simply knowing some facts about Him. It means knowing *Him*. There is a vast difference. You may be able to study all the available biographies of George Washington. As a result, you know a great deal about him. But you don't know him as, for example, Martha did. I may be able to tell you a great deal about someone who is a dear friend of mine, until at last you come to have as many facts as I can supply, but still that person is not thereby your friend — and could not be so until you came to know *him*. Just so, we can amass vast hoards of facts about God, and still not know *Him* — until we finally open our minds and hearts to Him in prayer and the sacramental life of the Church.

Until we come to know, we do not learn to love. I can be overwhelmingly infatuated by the girl of my dreams; but I cannot truly love her until I come to know her deeply. Then my love will be not just the high emotion of attraction, but the freely given choice of commitment, no longer

---

[26] Cf. *Instruction*, n.19.

40

dominated by the daily shifting of emotion. So, too, must we come to love God — loving Him not only in the frightening moments of need when we do not know where else to turn, nor only in the moments of fulfillment when we find our thanks so easy to express. To know Him fully is to love Him in every moment and in all ways. It is to love the One who made me, the One who keeps me alive, the One who leads me in the way I live.

To know and love God is also to serve Him. It is to come to realize that He does not ask what is impossible. He does not command what is useless. He demands only what is good — and that means not only good in the abstract, but good *for me*. Every commandment of God is geared to making me all that I was ever meant to be. To know and love Him is to long to know His will, for it is there alone that we find the fulfillment of all we yearn to be and to have. Seeking fulfillment anywhere else is an illusion.

All that we do in this world is, in the end, a choice for or against God. To choose against God is to choose nothing, because apart from Him we have nothing. Every commandment is saying simply, "Do this in order to find happiness." In the end, each time we reject the commandments, we reject our own happiness. That is what hell is all about. It is the rejection of God, the refusal to serve in love. The refusal to allow ourselves to be loved. It is to turn a blind eye, and a deaf ear.

It is quite clear that the kinds of choices we make about sex and reproduction and procreation are intimately linked to our love of God. This is why the Church sees it as so essential that it speak in these areas. What it offers is the light of revelation.

Each human being is special and unique in the eyes of God. Each one is loved by God, not as a faceless form in a jumbled mass of humanity, but as an individual, as *this* actual person. God does not simply know facts about me, He knows *me*. Each one is sacred and each one is called to the fullness of eternal life with God.

If we believe that we are not only bodies which live and finally sicken and die, but are also souls born for eternal life, then something else also follows. The creation of human life takes a special act of God in each instance, since there is no other way in which a spiritual and immortal soul can come to be. The start of a new human life is an act of God's creative love. This is also why human sexuality is so important and so sacred.[27]

There is in our freedom a frightening power as well. God has allowed us to share in His power to create life. The joining of egg and sperm is the moment in which God's love brings a human being into existence. That moment has been placed in our power also. We can procreate and we can kill. We can start the process and then abort it. We can start it in a petri dish and then use it, freeze it, destroy it or experiment with it.

Why does God allow it? Perhaps out of love. I am able to love or not, as I choose. If I do not love, then I begin a process of making choices which begin to hurt others, perhaps even to kill them. Could God end it right at the first by striking me dead or forcing me to change as soon as I take a step in that direction? I am sure He could. Does He? It certainly would seem not. He holds open to the end the chance for me to learn to love. I may come at

---

[27] Cf. Instruction, n.20.

last to the point where I will never change and then I am in hell. But God has not put me there. He has not destroyed me. I have done it to myself.

Could God have prevented my choices of evil, my failure to choose Him? He could, but not if He wants me to learn to love. If God calls us to be free in love, then even He cannot *force* us to do good. There is no such thing as love that is forced. Love must be chosen. If God makes us slaves to His will in order to prevent our evil choices, then love is gone. We are robots. God would be unfaithful to us and to Himself. Real love carries with itself the deepest sort of responsibility.

It is painful beyond measure to see a childless couple long for children, while around them babies are aborted. What does it do to them? There is no doubt that it tests their faith. That test does not come from God's failure to be good. It comes from human sinfulness. The sinfulness which kills the unborn reaches out and gets its grip on other innocent lives as well.

It is painful to see a childless couple become so intent on having a child, that they move slowly and surely to the point at which it seems they might do almost anything to have their dream fulfilled. There is nothing wrong with trying in many ways to correct what can be corrected. Some couples go to great trouble and expense in their efforts to be parents. Their virtue in this may be heroic, and it will have its reward.

It is dreadful to realize that their pain will also be met by those who will offer ways to have a child that will lead that same couple to do the very thing they so deplore. They may be offered the chance to look for "donors" of egg or sperm, and so be drawn to infidelity, after all that they have thus far done out of love for each other. They may be advised to try methods that produce and then discard the lives so created. They may be faced with methods which lead to multiple pregnancies and then are told that some must be killed — "selective reduction" it is named for purposes of sanitizing the process — in order for the others to live. Suddenly they are doing the very thing which caused their hearts to ache before.

What of those couples who try without success what can rightly be done, and then wait out the long period of pre-adoption? Their commitment to each other and to God and to what is right will make them both grow in holiness. Their support for each other will deepen their love. As, in love, they help each other through the times of doubt, their faith will grow. When, at last, they do become parents, their child will grow up knowing it is wanted. That child will be raised by parents who know what it is to be tempted almost beyond endurance, and yet to choose the right. They can be parents whose lives will be living examples of love and the fullest respect for life.

All that I have said emerges not just from reason, but from the love of God revealed to us and calling us to the greatest happiness and perfection. The *Instruction* points to all of this, hinting at it in a few short sentences, when it says: "From the moment of conception, the life of every human being is to be respected in an absolute way because man is the only creature on earth that God has 'wished for himself' and the spiritual soul of each man is 'immediately created' by God; his whole being bears the image of the Creator. Human life is sacred because from its beginning it involves 'the creative action of God' and it remains forever in a special relationship with the Creator, who is its sole end."[28]

Is it any surprise that, in view of this, we read: "Human procreation requires on the part of the spouses responsible collaboration with the fruitful love of God; the gift of human life must be actualized in marriage through the specific and exclusive acts of husband and wife, in accordance with the laws inscribed in their persons and in their union."[29]

It is clear enough why the society in which we live has so many problems with love and the real, lasting commitment of marriage. There is a clear effort to separate sex from its procreative function and to treat it *only* as somehow uniting the partners or even as no more than recreation. That takes away almost every trace of the sacred or of collaborating in the work of God. There is a blind eye, but it leads to no victory. It simply closes people to the real vision of their own worth.

The revelation of a saving and creative God also contains another implication. If human life is sacred and if each human being is truly loved by God, then we have the deepest sorts of obligations to each other. To say that we must love our neighbor as we love ourselves is not simply to mouth a platitude. It is a truth that must come to life in us if we are to be what we are meant to be and if we are to find real happiness.

In the end, the Lord of all life is God, not man. This is true from life's beginning to its end. "No one can, in any

---

[28] *Instruction*, n. 20.

[29] *Instruction*, n. 21.

circumstance, claim for himself the right to destroy directly an innocent human being."[30]

In some way, I suppose, such blindness should not totally surprise us, since it is a blindness to revelation and can be overcome only by faith — and for many that act of faith seems hard to come by.

There is, however, another kind of blindness as well. Human reason itself is ignored. I do *not* mean that it is hard to grasp, and therefore many cannot see it. I mean that there are those who are *willfully* blind to the acceptance of what reason can clearly and, indeed, easily prove. But many do *not want* to know, and they do all they can to keep others from finding out. They even sing the praises of science, but do it with their eyes tight shut, for fear that the truth might face them with the need to change. They hide and ignore the evidence, because all the evidence of science itself says that they are wrong.

To turn one blind eye is bad enough, but then to put a patch over the other is insane. To set aside both revelation and reason is to view ourselves and the world with two blind eyes. That leads only to failure.

---

[30] *Instruction*, n. 20.

# CHAPTER 8
## CONVERSATIONS WITH THE MAD HATTER

*Alice had been looking over [the Mad Hatter's] shoulder with some curiosity. "What a funny watch!" she remarked. "It tells the day of the month, and doesn't tell what o'clock it is!" "Why should it?" muttered the Hatter, "Does your watch tell what year it is?" "Of course not," Alice replied very readily; "but that's because it stays the same year for such a long time together." "Which is just the case with mine," said the Hatter. Alice felt dreadfully puzzled. The Hatter's remark seemed to her to have no sort of meaning in it, and yet it was certainly English.*[31]

In this and the next few chapters I will talk about the life of the unborn. The *Instruction* deals with this in terms of respect for the embryo, as a foundation for what will be said about diagnosis and therapy on the unborn. It is also a necessary foundation for what must be said later in regard to techniques in aid of procreation. It is on the same ground that judgments will be made about fetal research and experimentation.[32]

---

[31] Lewis Carroll, *Alice in Wonderland.*

[32] Cf. *Instruction*, n. 23.

Most people, of course, have heard all sorts of arguments, both pro and con. My intention in this and the next few chapters is to look at why the unborn child should be considered as human and why it should be treated as a person. Many of the arguments in favor of abortion are what I would call "Mad Hatter" arguments — those which sound like English but have, in fact, no real meaning. They are actually ridiculous arguments, but people hear them and think that perhaps they make some sense. One way to tell if arguments are worthwhile or not is to see where they really lead. If, in fact, they lead to stupid conclusions, then they are stupid arguments. These are "Mad Hatter" arguments.

I should also, I think, point out something else. I am *not* using the teaching of the Church as an argument against abortion. Rather, I will base my arguments on the clear and unarguable facts of science. I will respond to poor arguments in favor of abortion, *not* by saying they differ from Catholic teaching, but simply by pointing out what is wrong with the arguments themselves. The arguments in this chapter are, I would say, the most foolish, but they are given by people and so I shall respond to them.

**"Why is the Church against abortion? Don't they realize this is 1991?"**

What the date has to do with whether a thing is right or wrong is, I must admit, beyond me. If there were any sense to it at all, then every New Year's day should bring along with it a whole new set of rules. Each year everything would have to be reexamined. "What do you mean, robbery is illegal? This is 1991!" In fact, if time is what makes things right or wrong, then why even wait for a new year? "Of course I can murder you. It's three o'clock!"

Enough said. Even the Mad Hatter wouldn't take that argument very seriously.

Or do they mean that by 1991 we have learned enough to know that a fetus is not human? Well, if that's the case, then we should have no trouble finding out what that new knowledge is. But when we look at what science and medicine can tell us, we find just the opposite! Every new bit of information actually adds more evidence that a fetus is human. This we shall see perfectly clearly in the next few chapters.

**"It isn't human, at least not in the first few months. After all, it's not even an inch long."**

Short people, beware! If this argument is true, then it follows that the smaller we are, the less human we are. Or is there some magic size which determines our humanity? Six inches? A foot? Just as time is not a norm for making a thing right or wrong, so length is certainly not a norm for making us human. Of course, it may be hard for some people to realize just how so small a being can be human, or how we can tell that it is. That will all be explained in the following chapters. Right now I just want to point out that if you can honestly be convinced that length itself is the final answer, then sit down and let the March Hare pour you a cup of tea. The Hatter will enjoy talking to you.

**"It isn't really human, until it can live on its own, outside the uterus and independent of its mother."**

This argument may mean various things. First of all, some people may propose it with the idea that the fetus, before it is viable (that means being able to live outside the womb), is part of the mother's body and, therefore, not an individual being in its own right. People sometimes say this simply because of lack of information. They are surprised to learn that, no matter what else science may or may not be able to say about the fetus, the one thing that science can say truthfully, absolutely, positively and beyond all doubt is this: *The fetus is never, at any stage of its life, a part of the mother's body.* Never! It is, with no possibility of contradiction, from the moment of conception, clearly distinct from its mother. This point is so important that it deserves more than passing reference. I will explain it in some detail in the next few chapters.

The second meaning of the same argument is really the one that falls into the Mad Hatter category. They say that the total dependence of the unborn child on its mother means that it is not yet human. If it is the fact of dependence which is the issue, then the child is not human even after it is born. Even after birth the child still needs to be fed and clothed and sheltered. If left on its own, it will die. That helpless condition lasts for quite a few years. In fact, if you listen to what mothers say, then even some teenagers and an occasional helpless husband might not survive without a woman to take care of them. In other words, if we take seriously the idea that being human is determined by total independence, then we are all in trouble.

**"Up to 50% of all embryos do not implant in the uterus and just die spontaneously. There cannot be very much wrong with aborting them."**

First of all, although I have heard people use this argument and quote that statistic, I have never found one bit of evidence to support it. I don't really doubt that some eggs are fertilized, begin to develop, and are then unable (for whatever reason) to implant in the wall of the uterus. This would result in a very early miscarriage, of which a woman might not even be aware. But there is simply no evidence to tell us how often that actually happens.

50

What about the argument itself? It is utterly stupid to say that because some — even 50% — die, it is therefore all right to kill them. If the argument is a good and sensible one, then we should be able to say this: 100% of adults die, therefore it is perfectly all right to kill them.

**"The embryo is nothing but differentiated tissue. Therefore it is not human and can be aborted."**

Now here is a real one for the Mad Hatter. Some pro-abortionists used to say that the embryo was just *undifferentiated* tissue. This means there is just a mass of cells, all alike, no one different from another. However, that statement was simply not true, and they knew it. The cells are not alike. In fact, by the time the embryo reaches the uterus (just a few days after it is fertilized) it has already developed enough to have various sorts of cells. Some of them (called chorionic villi) are what make implantation possible.

Since they cannot truthfully say that it is undifferentiated tissue, some have begun to say that it is just *differentiated* tissue! This means it is a being composed of various kinds of specialized cells and organs! Well, so is an adult. If you can kill whatever is composed of differentiated tissue, then you can kill anyone. This might also fall into the category of arguments that even the Hatter would laugh at.

To conclude, I would point out again that when you can take an argument and honestly and logically follow it to ridiculous conclusions, then there is a real flaw in the argument. It is not true and it is no more than suitable conversation for the Mad Hatter.

# CHAPTER 9
## A PRETTY KETTLE OF FISH

I have never, I must admit, outgrown the pleasure of seeing those old Laurel and Hardy movies. Stan's injured innocence catapults them into one disaster after another, as Ollie bemoans his fate: "Another pretty kettle of fish you've gotten us into!" In fact, the same comment was made by Queen Mary to the Prime Minister of England when her son, Edward, abdicated the throne back in the 1930's. (I mean the comment about the kettle, not about liking Laurel and Hardy movies.).

Those kettles, I suppose, could contain just about any sort of fish, but some are worse than others. Among the most insidious are red herrings, and swallowing them is even worse than falling into the kettle.

No diet is more unhealthy for us than a good catch of red herrings. The resulting intellectual indigestion also has the effect of upsetting our ability to make good moral choices. The readers of many of our Sunday newspapers were recently treated to a noble feast of those elusive little creatures by Carl Sagan and Ann Druyan in an article that they wrote for *Parade Magazine*.[33]

---

[33] Carl Sagan and Ann Druyan, "Is it possible to be Pro-Life and Pro-Choice?" in *Parade Magazine*, April 22, 1990, pp. 4-8.

The whole menu was served up under the heading of "Science on Parade" due, I suppose, to the fact that Doctor Sagan, as a result of his public television *Cosmos* series, has become such a well known scientist. What was offered, however, was far from scientific. It was, in fact, a kind of pseudo-philosophizing which, in the end, ignored the scientific facts in favor of a dubious compromise to respect life and do away with it at the same time.

They start out, in a sense, on the right track. The newborn baby is a human person, even by legal definition. The legal absurdity, however, is that even one day before the birth of a third trimester baby our present laws, as interpreted by the Supreme Court's *Roe v. Wade* decision, would allow it to be legally aborted. It would not be accorded the rights of a person nor the full protection of the law. Yet the newborn child outside the womb is certainly not a different being than it was a day before or a moment before birth. Why is the act of killing the child considered as murder just after the birth, but not just before?

As they point out in their article, this is a question that should bother even those who are pro-abortion. It is so patently absurd. They are probably right in their assessment of the reason why pro-abortionists do not dwell on the topic. To do so would be to allow that the state has a right — even a duty — to intervene; and this might imply something they do not wish to accept. If we acknowledge the duty of the state to intervene at *any* time in the pregnancy, then we might have to accept that it ought to intervene in favor of the unborn at *all* times. That is what they want to reject.

The two authors make a passing comment, however, which will represent the attitudes of many people. They say that the question of third trimester abortions has little practical value, since no more than 1% of recorded abortions take place in the last three months of pregnancy. That does sound like a small number, until you recall that there are 1.6 million abortions a year in this country and that, therefore, third trimester abortions amount to 16,000 annually. Anything else that caused a yearly death rate of 16,000 would be considered a problem of major proportions. In fact, even if there were less than 1% it would not be insignificant, since we are dealing with human life.

In any case, Sagan and Druyan begin to focus on the question of just when we can say that the killing of a fetus is the killing of a human being. Here, too, they are focussing on the right issue. Unfortunately, it is at this point that the appetizer comes to an end and we start dipping from our pretty kettle of fish. They start by discussing what we mean when we speak of "right to life."

They begin by saying that no society on earth ever has accepted the concept of "right to life." Of course, they then go on to explain that this statement is based on the fact that plants and animals are killed as food and for all sorts of other reasons. Therefore, they conclude, we must be talking only about *human* life. Well, indeed we are. That should be no surprise to anyone, really. Plants and animals are not persons, and it is *persons* who have rights. It is cruel and inhuman to destroy animals wantonly, just as it is cruel and inhuman to inflict needless pain and suffering on them. This, however, is not because animals are persons with rights, but because that sort of cruelty is dehumanizing to its perpetrators and begins the process of internal self-destruction of their own human sensitivities.

Granted that we are speaking of human life, they then speak of the ways in which even human life is treated with disregard. Murder, war and starvation by neglect are part of

54

the news every day. Mass murders have been organized and carried out by governments who should have been in the business of protecting human life — although they have often enough tried to justify this by first attempting to show that their victims were somehow not truly human. There are millions of children who die by preventable causes every day.[34] The right to life has eluded them.

It should be pointed out that none of this argues against the real right to life. The right exists. What is lacking is the protection and respect, the care and concern, which would allow the right to be exercised. The question still comes down to what makes a human being unique and just when does a being become human, and it is to this point that Sagan and Druyan return.

They then begin to dole out another ladle of herrings. Life, they say, does not begin at conception. It is, rather, "an unbroken chain that stretches back nearly to the origin of the Earth." Human life dates back to the origin of our species. Somehow, this comes across as profound. My equally profound response would be, "So what?" We are not concerned with the origin of human life in this sense. We are concerned, rather, with the first moment of life of each *individual* human being. Indeed, the concept of "human life" as they are speaking of it here is an abstraction and it is a mistake in the most elementary sort of logic to confuse the abstract and the concrete.

Next they point out that every human sperm and egg is alive, but this does not mean that they are human beings. The sperm and egg, each carrying half of the genetic code

---

[34] They cite the statistic of 40,000 children under the age of 5 who die each day from preventable causes.

for a human being, must come together. They can, after fertilization and under the right circumstances, become a baby.[35] Therefore, they argue, neither a sperm and egg separately nor a fertilized egg is more than a *potential* baby or *potential* adult. Why then, if it is murder to kill a fertilized ovum, is it not murder to kill a sperm or an egg? This is no fast food red herring. This is the highest class of *paté de hareng saur*. It is herring mashed and seasoned and spread on little triangles of toast. It is also stupid, as is evidenced when they try to conjure up the image of a corps of sperm police trying to prove that masturbation is mass murder.

First of all, the sperm *by itself* or the egg *by itself* will never develop into a full human person. Either is a potential human being only in conjunction with the other. The fertilized egg, however, is quite another matter. If allowed to develop, it will indeed become a baby and, eventually, an adult. It will live its life from beginning to end, if allowed to. It is *potentially* a full term baby, only because it is *already* and *actually* a living being, an individual distinct from either of its parents. To say, as they do, that the egg and the sperm are as human as the fertilized ovum is nonsense. "Human cell" is not the same as "human being." Sagan and Druyan both know better than to imply that a germ cell is "as human" as an embryo — they know that the meanings are quite different.

They also argue that the most common reason for abortion is birth control, and, therefore, those who are opposed to abortion should be busy handing out contraceptives.

---

[35] They also make the thoroughly unsubstantiated statement that *most* fertilized eggs are spontaneously miscarried. There is no doubt that *some* are, but there is no evidence whatsoever that *most* are. Cf. supra, Chapter 8.

56

Another herring.    Contraception is a lesser evil than abortion, but that does not make it into a good.  What is needed is not contraception to prevent abortion, but a grasp of the sacredness of human sexuality to prevent both.  The person who is really pro-life should be dedicated to teaching the full meaning of human sexuality and should not be satisfied with finding some sort of mechanical or chemical short cut.

Sagan and Druyan go on next to the question of just when we become human. They point out the fact that the Christian tradition has frequently discussed this in terms of "ensoulment." This means the moment at which the human soul is first present.   As they indicate, the time of ensoulment has been explained differently at different times in history.  The reason for this is simple enough, but Sagan and Druyan do not go into any explanation.   Perhaps, however, they should not be too harshly criticized for this. They, like many people, may think that theologians just operate on some sort of abstract theological basis. The fact is that in this area especially theologians have consistently acted upon the basis of science.

Since the soul is not visible, we can only infer its presence or absence by observing its actions.[36]  The soul is the principle of human life, and so we can only see its actions insofar as we can observe the presence of human life. Before there was any possibility of observing the sperm or the egg, there were those who thought that the male seed contained human life itself.  It was placed in the woman's uterus at the time of intercourse and it was nourished by her blood.  This is logical enough if all you can observe is

---

[36] Further explanation of this will be given below, in chapter 12.

57

that pregnancy follows intercourse and during pregnancy the woman's menstrual flow ceases.

Later observers learned further facts. When they saw miscarried or aborted fetuses large enough to be visible to the eye, they also saw the changes which take place in the course of pregnancy. Without more modern tools for examination, the fetus is not easily discernible to the naked eye as human shaped until about the sixth week. Even then, at about 40 days or so, any fetus might appear to the naked eye as male. It is only later, as it approaches the ninth week, that sexual differentiation is clearly visible. Is it any surprise then that some medieval theologians — *and scientists* — would have thought that the human soul becomes present at about the fortieth day for boys and about the sixtieth day for girls? Nor is it shocking to realize that some speculated that the growing embryo went through stages where there might be a vegetative soul and then an animal soul and, finally, a human soul. They were attempting to learn, but their capacity for accurate observation was severely limited. When they then agreed that it is wrong to abort a human being, they also had different ideas as to just when the fetus was to be considered truly human.

It is actually modern science and modern methods of observation which have made it abundantly clear that there is but one life present from the very moment of conception and that such life is human. The full genetic code of human life becomes present at the moment when the egg is fertilized by the sperm. If, then, we say that a human being is not to be killed, we should realize that we are dealing with a human being from the moment of conception. The life of a new individual is there from the first and it need only be allowed to live in order to be able, step by step, to realize all of its potential activity. It is not a *potential* human being. It's an *actual* human being, potentially capable of all that a human being can be or do.

Sagan and Druyan contend that the fetus becomes truly human only when it is capable of characteristically human thought. This, they say, becomes possible only with the large scale linking of neurons in the brain at about the sixth month, and regular brain wave patterns similar to those of an adult come in the third trimester.

Rather than accept the observable continuity of human life from its conception, they prefer to look for "a developmental criterion" at which they can draw the line for abortion. This line they draw at six months, and so end up right in line with the 1973 *Roe v. Wade* decision.

When Sagan and Druyan come finally to evaluate the Court's decision in *Roe v. Wade*, they find it somewhat lacking. It is based on the woman's right of privacy in her "reproductive freedom." In the first trimester it is this "right" which is given precedence. The state's right to prohibit abortion is upheld in the third trimester, thus giving precedence to life. The criterion used by the Court is viability — the capacity of the child to live outside the uterus. The authors find this "a very pragmatic criterion." As they point out, the time of viability is, to a large extent, determined by the advances of technology. Placing the weight of moral decisions on so changeable a foundation is truly no more than the worst kind of pragmatism and it undermines any real objectivity in morality as a basis for the Court's decision.

All of this simply points out once more just how poor a decision was really made in *Roe v. Wade*. Whether that decision came from ignorance, stupidity, pragmatism or political pressure is hard to determine. In any case, it is clear that it did not come from objective criteria of either science or morality. It is glaringly arbitrary and never even addresses the issue of the fetus as person.

Since the issue of viability is so shaky as a criterion, Sagan and Druyan offer, in its place, the criterion of the earliest onset of human thinking. This they determine by the first instance of brain waves comparable to those of an adult. Since the capacity to think is characteristically human, they find it a better criterion than viability — which is based to a large extent on the capacity to breath air. Therefore, they would allow (with, it would seem, some reluctance) for abortion up to the time that brain waves may be first detectable. This would be in the third trimester. The result of their reasoning is that they declare *Roe v. Wade* to be a "good and prudent decision," even though it had been based on poor reasoning.

Unfortunately, the conclusion that they draw is also based on poor reasoning and is just as bad as the pragmatic *Roe v. Wade* decision. The brain, first of all, is present and functioning long before the third trimester. It does not yet emit *adult* brain wave patterns. But, then, do we expect a child to act as an adult? If we cannot expect the same physical or mental responses from a child already born, then we surely have no right to expect them from those not yet born. In neither case does this argue against the fact that they are human. It merely recognizes that human life in this world is a process, starting at conception and ending at death.

Their argument is every bit as arbitrary as was that of the Supreme Court. They have simply chosen the brain function at a certain level, in place of the capacity to breathe. In either case, what has been chosen is one definable point in a continuum of individual life. If their argument had any truth in it, then it could be used also to justify the killing of the newly born, since their brain waves — and, indeed, their conduct — do not yet show adult patterns.

When you try to judge the values of an argument, examine very carefully the conclusions you can draw from it. If the conclusions are wrong or stupid, then so is the argument. The argument given by Sagan and Druyan can be applied as well to some of those who are profoundly retarded. It can even be applied to certain people under the influence of central nervous system depressants, such as barbiturates, or to victims of hypothermia. In these cases you will not get normal adult brain wave patterns and you may even get a flat electroencephalogram, characteristic of no activity in the cerebral cortex. Does this mean that we are justified in killing such people on the ground that they are no longer human? Indeed it does not. In fact, in the latter two cases the victims may fully recover their normal brain functions. At the moment of examination, when such functions are not detectable, they are *potentially* capable of normal adult response. Given time, they can and frequently do come to that response. Yet the logical conclusion of Sagan and Druyan's argument is that they are at that moment not human. If they would say that they do not intend their argument to mean this, then the argument is a bad one.

Their argument is poor and their "compromise" is no compromise at all. It is the same old problem of finding a way to declare certain persons non-human so that we can get rid of them for reasons of our own. The fact is that, if people had no desire to do away with them, the "doubts" about their humanity would never even arise. As much as I like seafood, red herrings simply do not agree with me.

# CHAPTER 10

## BY THE LIGHT OF THE MOON

Someone who had been in Africa, in the Peace Corps, once told me a story about some tribal lore that he had heard there. Some of the people he had come across were convinced that the moon was much brighter than the sun. How, you may ask, did they ever come to that conclusion? It may surprise you to learn that their reasons were, to them, both logical and obvious. You can see the moon at night, even in the dark. You can see the sun only on clear, bright days. Where do you begin if you want to correct that source of misconception? It comes from a thorough confusion of cause and effect. It arises from a complexity of misinformation, and correction will have to begin with clear and accurate information.

Where do you begin with people who say that the fetus is not a human being, when their reasons for saying this are a hodge-podge of misinformation? It seems to me that we might best begin with the facts, apply them to what they say, and then see what comes of it.

**"The embryo or fetus is just formless tissue."**

Let's look at that and see just what the truth really is. I mentioned in the earlier chapter that a common argument for the pro-abortionists was that the embryo is just a bit of undifferentiated cells, a formless mass of tissue. I also said that this was certainly not true. Now I think it is time for me to offer some simple facts about what does happen within the uterus during a pregnancy. What I am going to say is really quite simple. I will describe what can be readily observed about a growing embryo. None of this is guesswork and any book on embryology will support what I say. If you would like to *see* what I am talking about, there are books, films and video tapes which you can get and which are listed in the footnote.[37]

At the moment of conception an egg (ovum) of the woman is fertilized by a sperm from the man. The head of the sperm enters into the egg, usually while it is moving along somewhere in the upper one-third of the fallopian tube (the tube leading from the ovary into the uterus). One sperm enters in and immediately the chemical composition of the outer layer of the egg changes, so that no other sperm can enter. The sperm and the egg each have 23 chromosomes, which give the fertilized egg a total of 46 — the normal total in every cell of a human being. In fact, once the ovum is fertilized it is no longer called an ovum. Instead, it is referred to as a *zygote*. It immediately begins a very rapid process of growth and specialization.

The zygote is still not attached to the body of its mother. For a week it continues its slow movement through the tube and by the end of that week it has become 150 cells, already forming the first organs that it will need in order to implant itself in the uterus. That implantation takes place in the second week of its life, and at that point it is no

[37] Mirjam Furuhjelm, Axel Ingelman-Sundberg, Claes Wirsén, (photographs by Lennart Nilsson), *A Child Is Born*, Delacorte Press/ Seymour Lawrence, 1980. *Nova: The Miracle of Life*, WGBH Boston, Crown Video, N.Y.,1982 (60 Minute Color Video Tape). *The First Days of Life*, 16mm Film, McGraw-Hill Films (about 30 Minutes).

longer referred to as a zygote. It is now called, instead, an *embryo*.

The embryo is far from formless tissue. It is quite well formed indeed. When it first implants it looks a bit like a ball covered with hairlike appendages called *villi*. These are what reach into the lining of the uterus and hold on. The process of forming complex and specialized organs and functions never ceases. By the end of its third week of life (when the mother is just realizing that she has missed a period and may be pregnant) its heart has begun to beat. A week later (when its mother may be deciding to go to a doctor for a pregnancy test) there is a nervous system, a functioning brain and the beginnings of eyes and ears. Yet it still has some 36 weeks to go before it is ready for full term delivery.

When the embryo is only eight weeks old, it is already complete in all its essential organs and is now referred to as a *fetus*. What began as one living cell is now a collection of tens of thousands of cells. They are absolutely *not* formless. All the parts and organs are in place and operating under the direction of the brain. The fetus at this point is just over an inch long — about the length of the first joint of your thumb. It is clearly human even to simple observation — head, body, legs, arms, hands and feet.

Many people speak of pregnancy as being divided into trimesters — three periods of three months each. The Supreme Court, in its sad *Roe v. Wade* decision of 1973, allowed anyone to elect to have an abortion in that first trimester. Their decision certainly left many with the impression that the fetus in those first three months had no claim to be called human. Did you ever wonder if the justices who rendered that decision knew very much about anatomy? I suspect that they know as much about anatomy as most doctors know about law — and that may not be much at all. Did they ever look at pictures of what they were talking about? I have some doubt about it. Yet they said it could be aborted and that the government had no compelling interest in the protection of its life.

You perhaps noted above that when I described the fetus as complete with all its organs, I was speaking of it during its eighth week of life. That is a whole month before the end of the first trimester! It is still too small for its mother to feel its movements, but it is already moving its arms and legs and living its life.

By the twelfth week of life (as it comes to the end of the first trimester) it has grown to be three inches long (about the size of your little finger). The organs and body parts are growing rapidly and will continue to grow and become more refined — *but no new parts are added.* They have all been there since the eighth week.

The fetus has been moving ever since its seventh week of life, but it has been so small that its mother has not been able to feel it. She will be aware of it by the time it is about six inches long. By then it will be sixteen weeks old. About this time also it is beginning to react to light and sound and taste. Its senses are in quite good working order.

Growth and movement and response all continue. By its twenty-fourth week of life the fetus is self-aware and responds even to the sounds of voices, especially the voice of its mother. In fact, there is some speculation that this may even be the first stage of its ability to learn language. It has not yet reached the end of the second trimester, but it is now just at the earliest point of viability.

It is at the twenty-fourth week, or just before that, that its lungs are at the stage where it would be able to breathe. Of course, if it were born this early it would need a great deal of special care and assistance. Every day of the remaining sixteen weeks of pregnancy will find it growing stronger and being more and more able to leave the warmth and safety of the womb. Each day makes its survival increasingly easy and secure.

The final three months in the womb are a time of added growth and strengthening. The child gets more baby fat and is prepared for birth. When that moment arrives, that one cell of nine months ago will have become a complex, wonderful human baby of some 6,000,000,000,000 cells.

How did it all come about? From the first moment of its existence it was a living being, gradually becoming more and more complex and increasingly able to live with less and less total support from its mother. Even after birth that same process will continue. In other words, it really is nonsense to make the moment of birth appear to be the start of real human life, when it is plain as the nose on your face that it is one continuous process from beginning to end.

Please note something else also: Everything that I have said is based not on some obscure point of doctrine or faith. It is all based, rather, on simple observation of what really happens. You can read about it in a book on embryology. You can see it in some of the extraordinary films that are now available.

To say that the embryo is ever just a formless piece of tissue is absolute nonsense. But people do say so. Why? I am sure that many times they are merely repeating what they have been told. They have not been given a chance to learn the facts. That, in my opinion, is sad. People choose abortion at times without being told the truth. They talk about informed consent and free choice. But consent is never informed unless there is information communicated. Without it we can only give the consent of ignorance, and that certainly leaves one no chance at all for any sort of truly responsible freedom.

There are those, of course, who have heard or seen enough to begin to grasp the truth. But they may not want it. Closing our eyes to the truth is quite irresponsible — especially when it results in the death of someone who is given no choice at all in the matter. This sort of irresponsibility is, of course, far worse than simple ignorance.

There is, however, something even worse. The statement that an embryo is just a formless piece of tissue, is not true. When that statement comes from a doctor or a nurse or an abortion counselor, it is damnable. If they think they are telling the truth, then they are guilty of criminal ignorance and they ought to be drummed out of business as quacks and charlatans. They are worse than sellers of snake oil and bogus cures for disease. At least those people may avoid doing any real harm. The abortionists kill people. On the other hand, if they say that the embryo is formless tissue, and all the while they really know better, then they are simply liars. In either case I wouldn't put any stock at all in their advice.

Why, you may ask, would they lie? What do they have to gain? The answer is simple. Money. Where else can a doctor of only mediocre ability earn a quarter of a million dollars a year in his spare time, and feel successful when every one of his operations ends with at least one person dead? If they ever stopped lying they would be out of business, but moonlighting as an abortionist is all too lucrative to abandon — even at the expense of human life.

# CHAPTER 11

# KINDERGARTEN COUNSELING

You feel unwell. You suffer from stomach pains. Where do you go for good advice? I presume you would go to a doctor. He will examine you and may find that you have an ulcer. If so, he gives you the proper medication, he gets you started on a better diet and, perhaps, on a better way of coping with stress. I can't imagine anyone in his right mind going to a kindergarten class and seeking advice from the students. They might tell you, "You have a pain in your tum-tum. Take some green pills or maybe some red ones and have a peanut butter and jelly sandwich and a glass of grape Kool-Aid."

It's a silly example. After all, who would look for such important advice from someone who was not in any way an expert on health? You wouldn't trust important decisions to people not equipped to make them. Or would you? How many people seek advice from those who know next to nothing? "My friend told me, and her aunt used to be a nurse, so she ought to know." Really? Or do you make decisions on the basis of something you saw on the news on television or read in the newspaper?

I remember during one of the papal elections (I think it was that of Pope John Paul II), I was watching the coverage on television when they announced that a Pope had been elected. One of the commentators — on a major network — described the excitement of the crowd, and part of his description was the astonishing statement that, "One of the Sisters in the crowd is so excited, that she is waving her cassock over her head." First of all, Sisters don't wear cassocks, priests do. Furthermore, if she *had* been wearing one and began waving it over her head she might have felt a bit chilly — or gotten arrested for indecent exposure.

To anyone familiar with the word "cassock" that man's comment was silly beyond belief. But he didn't think so. He was perfectly serious. It was just that he didn't know what he was talking about. It certainly made me stop and think. I would presume that the network didn't just pull in someone off the street to do that commentary. They surely assigned someone who was *supposed* to know what he was about and could have been presumed to have done some homework. He certainly spoke with the tone of absolute self-assurance — but he still didn't know what he was talking about.

How much of what I hear on the news or read in the papers can I take at face value? If they can be wrong in one area, and still sound so certain, why not in others as well? Or am I being too harsh over a little slip of the tongue? Well, I certainly wouldn't make a federal case out of that particular error — it was a bit stupid, but hardly of any great significance. But it does make me think.

Another, more substantial, example came up just after the release of the *Instruction* about which I am writing. On a Sunday afternoon just after that, one of the news shows dealt with it. Three reporters conducted interviews with theologians and asked them a number of questions. One of the nationally known reporters asked a question something like this: "If *in vitro* fertilization is sinful, then isn't the Church really saying that a child conceived in this way is born in sin and is therefore condemned?"

I suppose some people would have thought that was a highly perceptive and tough question. To very many the answer would be obvious: Of course a child is not guilty because of a sin of its parents. There was, however, an interesting factor involved. In the document itself it says: "Although the manner in which human conception is achieved with IVF [*in vitro* fertilization] and ET [embryo transfer] cannot be approved, every child which comes into the world must in any case be accepted as a living gift of the divine Goodness and must be brought up with love."[38] In other words, the reporter had clearly *not* done his homework very well. He was asking questions on a document that he had either not read or whose clear words he had not understood.

My point is that news programs, even when done with such self-assurance and such a feeling of authority, may be full of real misinformation or serious lack of understanding. Yet so many people base even life or death situations on what they hear or read, and mistakenly think that they are getting the truth. There is also in the media a definite anti-Church and pro-abortion bias. Even when this is not fully conscious, it still colors the reporting.

**"A woman has rights over her own body. Therefore she has the same rights over the life of the fetus since it is part of her body and not a separate human being."**

We are told this over and over again. We see one reporter after another who either accepts this as true, or who doesn't seem to challenge it when he hears it said. Nonetheless, it is absolutely false. Medical personnel who say that it is true are simply lying. If they know even

---

[38] *Instruction*, n. 84.

70

elementary embryology, then they know full well that an embryo is *never* a part of its mother's body.

In the normal course of events, a woman's body will release one mature ovum each month. Her left and right ovaries take turns, so each one produces just one ovum every other month. The ovum grows inside a sort of cavity, a hollow called a follicle. When the egg is ripe, the follicle bursts and the ovum is ejected onto the surface of the ovary. The end of the fallopian tube looks like a piece of fringe (*fimbria*), and its movement guides the egg into the tube. The egg is, of course, inside the woman's body, but is not attached to it. It enters the tube and is gently moved along toward the uterus. It is somewhat like an object flowing in a stream, moved along by the flow, but distinct from the stream itself.

If the egg is not fertilized, it will move on into the uterus and be washed away in the menstrual flow as the uterine lining breaks down and prepares for the next month.

If the egg is fertilized (usually in the upper one-third of the tube), then the lining of the uterus will not break down and the zygote (the fertilized egg) will implant itself in the wall of the uterus, in tissue which is thick and rich with blood vessels to supply nourishment.

How does the woman's body know whether the lining is supposed to break down or not? It is due to the zygote, which immediately begins its own activity, *its own life.* Before it ever implants, while it is still moving along freely in no way attached to its mother's body, it produces a chemical (called chorionic gonadotropic hormone) which gets into the mother's system and signals certain cells in the ovary to produce the hormones necessary for pregnancy. It is, in fact, the very first communication of this new living being with its mother.

It is an already complex and highly developed embryo which arrives in the uterus and implants itself there. "Aha!" you may say. All along I have been saying that the embryo is *never* a part of its mother's body. Yet here I am saying that it *implants* itself into the lining of the uterus. The fact is that implantation does *not* make it a part of its mother's body.

A plant, growing in the earth, depends on that earth for its life. If it is uprooted and pulled out of that earth, it will die. But it is clearly not a part of the earth, even though it grows there. As roots enter the soil and anchor the plant there while it draws up nourishment, so do the villi of the embryo anchor it in the thick, rich tissue of the uterine lining (the endometrium). The two *never* become one.

Another way to picture the relationship is to compare it to the interlaced fingers of two hands clasped together. They are joined, but they never become just one hand, nor does one ever become a part of the other.

There are also other ways to show that the embryo is not a part of its mother's body. If a geneticist examines the cells of an embryo, they are easily and clearly defined as *human* cells. If he examines the cells of the mother, he will, with equal ease, identify them as human. But if he compares the cells of the embryo with the cells of the mother, he can show beyond all doubt that they are not the cells of the same person. They are from two distinct individuals. Each has its own genetic code, and neither is the same as the other.

There is also something else of which some people are not aware. If you were to take some cells from the embryo and attempt to transplant them into the body of its own mother, in an effort to make them into one being, her body will immediately begin a rejection reaction and attempt to eject the embryonic tissue as foreign. There is no doubt whatsoever. They are two distinct human beings, and neither one is a part of the other.

There is, however, one more question that might be asked. Don't they have a common blood supply in order for the embryo to take in nourishment from its mother? Absolutely not! The two individual systems flow through their own sets of veins and arteries. The baby's blood is pumped by its own heart through its body and also through the umbilical cord into the placenta (where the embryo is attached to the wall of the uterus). It is there that the two blood systems run side by side, but without ever mixing. Nourishment, oxygen and waste are passed back and forth through the thin walls of the system, but there is no mingling of blood. It should be pointed out also that, if by accident the two blood systems do mix, there may in some cases be serious problems as each system treats the other as foreign.

There are, of course, those who will accept the fact that the child is not a part of its mother's body. But they will argue their right to kill it by saying that it is a "parasite" living off its mother, and a woman has a right to rid herself of it. It is a sad society which could even accept an argument such as that, yet we live in a time when there are all too many — even otherwise very good people — who define children as a burden rather than a gift. It is only a society such as that which could ever think of a child at its most helpless stage of life as a parasite.

None of what I have said is a matter of philosophy or theology or faith or theory or speculation. It is simple, provable, accurate, scientific fact. There is no doubt at all about any of it. There is no point in its whole existence at which the embryo can be honestly spoken of as being a part of its mother's body. Has anyone ever told you differently? If so, then that person was either a sort of kindergarten counselor, who didn't know what he was talking about, or a liar. In either case, watch out and don't put your trust there.

# CHAPTER 12

# QUACK, QUACK!

You see a man walking down the street with an animal on a leash. It has white feathers, a flat beak, big yellow feet, a pronounced waddle and, as it plods along, it says, "Quack, Quack!" With careful attention to every detail, and using all the hidden powers of your intellect, you conclude that it must be a French poodle.

If you can do this and stick to your conclusion no matter what evidence is brought forth, then you can begin to enter into the minds of those who support abortion. Ignore all proof, block out any hint of whatever may make you think, don't even look at the facts. Insist that things are the way you want them to be whether they are or not. Make an absolutely blind act of faith in the party line.

If you can get yourself into this frame of mind, then you can open up to yourself whole new vistas of possibility. You can enjoy depersonalized, irresponsible, shallow sex, with no regard for yourself, your partner or the consequences. You can ignore some of the deepest values in life and enjoy a carefree existence — provided you can stop worrying yourself about the fact that you may have to kill someone now and again.

I fully realize that there are some mothers who are led to abort their children through fear or near despair or pressure. They may even know that it is wrong, but there is no one to support or help them. To them we must give compassion and all the practical help we can provide. To them the strong statements above do not apply. But they do apply to those who offer abortion as the solution and to those who promote it and draw people into it. Those who ignore all evidence and insist on a purely legal right to kill the unborn.

### "The fetus is not human; it's not a person."

No one finds it good to live with guilt. When we feel it, we want to get rid of it. Some people have what might be called a "guilt complex." They feel a vague, or even a rather pronounced, sense of guilt even though they have done nothing wrong. People who feel this way need some counseling, perhaps, to help them to overcome their own fears or poor self-image. There are, of course, others who have another kind of guilt. They really have done or are doing something wrong. Their sense of guilt is quite a healthy response to reality. They don't need counseling just to rid themselves of an uncomfortable feeling. What they need is to quit doing the things they are doing and, probably, to make some amends for what they have already done.

There are those, of course, who are doing something wrong and want to get rid of the guilt without making any change in what they are doing. The only way they can manage that is to suppress their sense of right and wrong, or find a way to rationalize what they are doing, so that they can say that it is all right even when it isn't.

If you are involved in abortion, and if abortion is the murder of a human person, then you will feel tremendous guilt — and rightfully so. It takes no effort at all to find out that in an abortion you are killing something that is alive. Those who perform abortions and see a struggling fetus know that it is a living thing. Even the twitching pieces of a fetus chopped to bits by a suction pump are

76

quite clearly undergoing the final struggle of something that has been alive. It is possible, however, to try to feel better about it all if you can at least convince yourself that even if it was alive, it was not really a person. In the following paragraphs I would like to do what I can to remove that rationalized bit of false consolation.

What makes a human being a person? One answer is the presence of a human soul. Of course you can't see a soul. You don't know by direct observation when it arrives or when it is gone. You simply don't see it. Then how do you know when it is present? The answer is that you recognize its presence by its actions.[39]

When you are inside a room looking through a window on a windy day, how do you know that the wind is there? You can't see it. From inside the house you can't feel it. You may not even be able to hear it. But you can see what it does. Leaves move, trees sway, light objects are tossed about. You have no doubt at all that there is a wind. Indeed, you *know* that there is. This way of knowing is called inference. The presence of one thing leads you to infer the existence of another — a perfectly valid way of arriving at the truth. The fact is that science does this all the time. The study of subatomic particles is a perfect example. No one has ever seen them, but their actions have been observed and so we know that they are there.

If we say that death is the separation of body and soul, then how do we know when the soul has left? By infer-

---

[39] Cf. *Instruction*, nn. 25-26. In the text, I am not trying to reduce the question to a discussion on the human soul. I am concerned, rather, with the simple fact that all signs point to the presence of *human life* from conception. If that is so then one cannot say that there is life, but no human soul; and there are those who do indeed argue in favor of abortion in that way.

ence, of course. Every test designed to enable a doctor to declare that a patient really is dead is a matter of inference. What does the physician look for? There is no sign of vital activity — no movement, no spontaneous breathing. There is no reaction to external stimuli, even painful stimuli. The pupils of the eyes are fixed and dilated. They do not respond to even a bright light. All of these are signs that the brain is not functioning. None of the organs are doing what they are supposed to do. There is, of course, no growth. All *signs* of life are gone. The inference is that life is gone. The soul is gone.

How do we know that the soul is present? There is life. There is internal activity. There is growth. The organs of the body are functioning. The brain and the central nervous system are operating. If nourishment is supplied and the ordinary conditions for survival are met, then life will go on. If the life in question is that of a fertilized egg and it is not destroyed, then it will become an embryo. the embryo will become a fetus, then an infant, a child, an adolescent and, finally, an adult.

There is one unified, continuous and inevitable process. There is one living being from beginning to end. There is one life principle, one soul. There is, in other words, one living individual.

When we think of a being as a person, we usually think in terms of the power to know and love. In the fetus that *power* is present, since the fetus is human. It is, however, not yet being exercised, since the full capacities to do so are still in process of completion. There are stages in the growth and life of any human being at which the power exists but is not able to be used for one reason or another. Some will argue that the fetus is not yet able to relate in that knowing and loving way and therefore is not human;

78

not a person and so can be killed. This is another stupid argument, because it leads to a stupid conclusion. If it is true that a human being is only a person when able to respond in a knowing and loving way, then we should be able to justify killing people who are comatose or unconscious or very deeply asleep. Indeed, why not just as easily kill the profoundly retarded? Or even the anesthetized?

What has happened in society in the last few years? Many people have adopted a very stupid position — a position that history should cause us to view with enormous alarm. They have decided that religion should not be the arbiter as to who is or is not a person. This is related, perhaps, to a lack of faith in our culture. It is also, no doubt, related to an attitude which tends in general to reject religion as "quaint" or antiquated, when in reality it is a simple desire to try to ignore the moral demands that the living of religion entails. But they have decided that all the findings of science should be ignored also, even though science can establish beyond any doubt that an embryo is a living human being. They have said, instead, that we shall decide *by legal decree* who is or is not a human person. In other words, they have decided to ignore all available evidence and just make a proclamation instead. This is nothing but the worst kind of blind dogmatism. It comes down to the frightening statement that a human being will be considered a person only if civil government decides that it has an interest in preserving its life.

I have spoken in earlier chapters of the fact that arguments which lead to stupid conclusions are stupid arguments. This one is not only stupid, it is deadly. I am not just spinning a theory about this. I am actually able to point to the most horrible kinds of conclusions that have already come about from exactly this same attitude.

It always makes the pro-abortion people angry and nervous when you compare them to Hitler. I am about to do exactly that, and without apology. It is not a mean or unfair comparison. It is a simple matter of fact. Why did the people of Germany not rise up in protest when more than 6,000,000 Jews were imprisoned and then murdered or used for experiments? Because they were gradually led to accept this as justifiable. The Jews were presented as a threat to the life and economy of the country. They were a drain on its resources. They were valueless. Finally, by legal decree, they were no longer considered persons. The state had no compelling interest in preserving their lives. Their murder was legal. It may have been distasteful, but it broke no laws. In fact, if they were to be killed anyway, why not at lest make their death useful to society? Why not use them for experiment to advance the cause of genetic research and medical progress?

Babies are a burden. They threaten the welfare of parents and the economy of the country. They are cheaper to kill than to keep. They are not persons, by legal decree. We are free to kill them. It may be distasteful, but it breaks no laws. In fact, if they are to be killed anyway, why not get some use from their deaths by using them for research? The arguments are totally parallel. There is precisely the same attitude in both cases.

Can our courts be wrong in so basic and serious a matter? Is it possible that a nation founded on the right to "life, liberty and the pursuit of happiness," could simply decide that certain categories of human beings are "non-persons"? Could the Supreme Court itself take such a step if it were really so blatantly stupid a step as I have painted it to be? Are not the Justices more intelligent than that?

It is hard to escape the conclusion that one of two things happened. The first is that a group of otherwise intelligent men are so ignorant of the basic realities of the science of embryology that they have made an outstandingly stupid decision that cries out for correction. The second is that their attitudes were so biased in favor of abortion that they blinded themselves to the truth and made a decision so morally wrong that it still cries out for correction. Blind Justice was being served by blind Justices. Either thought is deplorable. Is it possible that any group of judges could be so dreadfully wrong?

It does not seem to me that we have been in the habit of appointing stupid persons to be Justices of the Supreme Court. Their appointments, of course, are highly political, but there are just enough safeguards in the system to preserve us from serious incompetence. This does not mean, however, that all of those who become Justices of the Supreme Court are equally capable, nor does it mean that each group of Justices is thereby preserved from making enormous blunders which will have to be faced and rejected by later courts. This is obvious in the fact that there have, indeed, been instances of reversal. There was one judgement that was so seriously wrong that its reversal came about not through a peaceful judicial process, but through a long and bloody civil war.

The American Civil War was fought for a variety of reasons, but there is no doubt that one of the reasons was slavery. Not only was it one reason among many, it was the one which captured the imagination of people and gave them a moral incentive to fight. It was one of the reasons why the European nations were unwilling to come to the aid of the South. Most civilized countries had abandoned the slave trade and abolished slavery. Yet this "peculiar institution" still existed in the southern half of the United

States, and even to this day we feel its prejudicial effects. No sane person today would argue in favor of it and no Supreme Court would dare to declare it legal.

Not so in 1857. On March 6 of that year, in the case of a slave named Dred Scott, the Supreme Court ruled once and for all that black people were not to be considered as human "persons" within the framework of the Constitution of the United States. Slaves were considered legal property to be bought, sold or killed at the discretion of the owner. They had no *legal* rights as persons — and that meant, of course, that they had no legal protection of any *moral* rights as persons. The parallels between the Dred Scott decision in 1857 and the *Roe v. Wade* decision in 1973 are startling:

Those who opposed slavery protested, but were met with the retort: "So you oppose slavery? It is against your moral, religions, and ethical convictions? Well, you don't have to own a slave, but don't impose your morality on the slave owner. He has the right to choose to own a slave. The Supreme Court has spoken. Slavery is legal..."

Then on January 22, 1973, the U.S. Supreme Court finally decided a very vexing question... [T]he court ruled once and for all that unborn humans were not legal "persons" according to the U.S. Constitution...

Those who opposed abortion protested, but were met with a retort that seemed an echo of slavery days. "So you oppose abortion? It is against your moral, religious, and ethical convictions? Well, you don't have to have an abortion, but don't impose your morality on the mother (the owner). She has the right to choose to have

82

mock horror if anyone presents a photograph of an aborted child. It is not even horror at the sight of a dead child. It is simply the horror of the pseudo-compassionate who in fact would not want a pregnant woman to see a picture of what is inside of her and how cruelly it can be destroyed. Facts are not only ignored, they are wilfully suppressed.

Abortion is categorized as a medical procedure. In our society we consider it criminal to perform any serious medical procedure on a person who has not been given *informed* consent. This means that you have a *right* to know what is being done, how it is to be done, what its results are and what side-effects you may expect as a result. If someone lies to you in the process of getting your consent, they are legally liable and you can take them to court. We have all heard of women who had abortions and were told beforehand that it was just a matter of removing formless tissue from the body. Anyone who was told that was being told a lie in order to gain their consent. I see no reason why that could not be made the basis of a perfectly valid suit which could be won in court. The person who told them that has to be either a liar or a total incompetent.

Abortion counseling done by pro-abortionists is a farce. It does not consist in telling the truth so that a woman can be helped or supported in making a choice of real alternatives. Rather, it consists simply in giving her enough distorted information to make her feel better about having an abortion. Why? Because if she doesn't have the abortion she will go instead to a real doctor and the abortionist will lose his money.

In the preceding chapters we have looked at an abundance of facts — real facts — all of them true, none of them theory or guesswork. From the moment that a human egg is fertilized, it begins to grow and develop. With astonishing speed it has a heart, a circulatory system, a nervous system and a brain.

From the first moment it is alive and self-contained. It depends on someone else for life; but don't we all in one way or other? Yet even in our greatest moments of dependence on others, we do not cease to be ourselves. Neither does an embryo. From the first it has its own life and it is never just a part of its mother's body. In fact, it is truly never a part of her body at all. It has its own unique genetic code, its own identity. Only poor scientific procedure, sloppy thinking, malice, love of profit or downright stupidity could confuse the identity of this unique being with another.

How many women who undergo abortion are told that within the embryo there is a beating heart and a functioning brain? By the time abortions are performed — even the earliest ones, in the first trimester — there is a clearly recognizable human being. And I don't mean recognizable only to a scientist, but to anyone who cares to look.

Recognizing that the embryo is a person is not a matter of faith. It is a simple use of human reason. You have, beyond all shadow of doubt, a living, growing, human individual. To conclude that it is not a person does violence to our intelligence. Indeed, why would the question even be brought up? There is only one reason, really. To be able to kill it without feeling bad about it. The only motive for claiming that it is not a person is that there are those who would *prefer* that it not be a person. The pro-abortionists must make a blind act of faith and be willing to protect their minds from the facts.

If we draw from all of this even the minimal conclusions, then we have to say at the very least that the human being, from the moment of conception, must be accorded the

88

rights due to every human person. Most basic of all is the simple right to be allowed to live. This is a *right* and it is not undone or outweighed by what many now like to speak of as a woman's "reproductive rights." Here is another catch word, another sanitized term misused to help hide the truth. (I sometimes think that we should gather all these terms together into a dictionary of abortion terminology. It could be sold wrapped in one of those "Sanitized for your Protection" ribbons that they wrap around the toilet seats in hotels.)

Are there such things as "reproductive rights"? Of course there are. The state should not be able to force an individual to reproduce. Nor should the state be able to intervene in the lives of its citizens to the extent that it can force them not to reproduce (as is being done, for example, in China). People should not be mated or bred like animals, being forced to reproduce with one partner or another. Indeed we do have reproductive rights. Unfortunately, the term is now being used to mean, "Having failed to use my reproductive rights in a responsible way, I now would like to kill my offspring."

Both men and women have rights over their own reproductive faculties. But rights are seldom absolute. They involve obligations and responsibilities. I cannot simply exercise a right without regard for its effect on others. If you don't think that holds true in the area of reproductive rights, then consider this: Can a rapist defend himself in court on the grounds that he was merely exercising his reproductive right? I sincerely hope not. He has no right at all to subdue or terrorize or harm or have sexual relations with a woman against her will on the ground that he is exercising his "reproductive rights." Rights have limits and those limits are defined by one's responsibilities not to violate the rights of others. The rapist is a criminal because he is guilty of such a violation. Neither can a woman be offered the false consolation of appeal to reproductive rights as a justification for killing an unborn child with rights of its own. Indeed, so basic a right as the right to life is not ours because the state grants it. It is ours by basic natural and moral law, and the state has no justifiable power at all to allow any of us to violate that right in any innocent person. Laws allowing or encouraging or paying for abortions are wrong, immoral, unjust and in violation of the most basic principles of civil government.

The true exercise of "reproductive rights" begins with the responsible use of sex. In fact, if people were honest with themselves, they would see that this is the real heart of most of the problem. They want "reproductive rights" but they are unwilling to face the fact that sex is and should be a reproductive faculty. Their use of sex is frequently as irresponsible as the way in which a child uses a real loaded gun as a toy. In either case, people get killed.

Another argument that is so often linked with that of a woman's "reproductive rights," is the statement that "it is her body and no man has the right to direct her use of it." Of course no man, merely because he is a man, has the innate right to tell a woman what to do, merely because she is a woman. That is nonsense, and it's something we should all get over. But when any of us, men or women, see serious evil being done, we must say something — out of respect for ourselves, if even for no deeper reason. The argument is a ridiculous caricature, trying to create the impression that it is men (nasty things) who are opposed to abortion and women (freed from foolish restriction) who are in favor of it. Utter nonsense.

Just look at who is involved on either side — men and women. It is not a man vs. woman issue, no matter how much some would like to create that impression.

It is nonsense to say that this is purely a woman's business. It is not women who are being killed by abortion (except, of course, for those victims of abortion clinics who suffer complications and are listed as dying from infection or hemorrhage — never from abortion). It is children who are being killed — male and female — and in that we all have an interest. It is an issue in which we should stop shouting slogans and begin looking at facts. If anything, it is an issue of truly responsible and loving sexuality on the one hand, and sex for fun and damn the results on the other. Did you ever notice that so many who favor abortion on demand would like to say that it has all emerged from men's "sex for fun" attitude and women's "responsible loving" response? Not so. Either gender can be found on either side. Don't let the rhetoric fool you.

Keep coming back to the facts. The unborn child is alive. It has rights. It is wrong to kill it. Its rights give rise to our corresponding obligations. Life is too precious and too sacred to be ignored. The facts are too clear and far too important to ignore.

# CHAPTER 14

# TELL ME WHERE IT HURTS

The first step in diagnosis is simple: Just tell me where it hurts. That, however, is rarely ever enough. The description of symptoms is usually followed by examination, which may become quite complex and demand the use of some rather elaborate techniques.

In the case of the unborn, the initial question may not even be possible. The child cannot answer and the mother may not be aware of any symptoms. In this case diagnosis will almost always involve some sort of intervention which may be quite invasive (e.g. amniocentesis) or relatively non-invasive (e.g. ultrasonography).

It is, in fact, now possible to intervene in the life of the child in the womb in a bewildering variety of ways, and for a sometimes equally bewildering variety of reasons. The *Instruction* categorizes those reasons under four general headings. Diagnostic, therapeutic, scientific and commercial.

Diagnosis is the art of determining if anything is wrong with a patient's health and, if so, discovering exactly what that condition is. It may have to make use of tools and techniques that can cause pain, some damage or even serious side effects. How free are we to use such methods on the unborn, who are unable either to express a need or give consent?

Therapy is the art of treating and, perhaps, healing diseases or disorders. Its obvious intent is certainly good, but its necessary use of drugs or technology may result in undesirable side effects. How are we to know what moral justification we have for the use of therapies that are in themselves dangerous or experimental? Even well informed adults may experience real anguish in making such decisions in reference to themselves. How are we to know what decisions to make on behalf of the unborn?

The "scientific" purpose of intervention is to acquire knowledge. That may prove quite beneficial. There are certainly moral limits as to how far one can go in involving adults in an experiment — even when those adults are well informed of all aspects of what will take place. There may well be risks. In areas of diagnosis or therapy, one can justify the taking of some risk, with the ultimate goal of regaining reasonably good health. In fact, the more life threatening a condition is, the greater risks we might be able to justify in fighting it. But what if the experiment is to be performed on someone who is not in need of therapy? How great a risk is he morally justified in taking? How are such decisions to be made for the unborn?

Commercial goals are those related to profit. No human being should ever be reduced to becoming a means of financial gain. This should not be done even if its victim seems willing. Surely it should be unthinkable to use the unborn in such a way? Think again. They have been and are now being used by some in exactly that way. There is a ready market for babies, both living and dead.

In each of these areas there are moral decisions to be made, as well as medical. Making those decisions means looking quite clearly and carefully at all sorts of possible medical procedures and their motives. It means looking at various implications and results. In fact, our moral responsibility extends through the whole process, and it never suffices to claim that our intentions were good if we initiate a process that results in something morally evil. It is all further complicated by the fact that we are concerned with the unborn who cannot yet make a decision about any of this.

For the moment I would like to look particularly at the question of diagnosis. We can consider some general principles and then apply them more specifically in the coming chapters. Although I will save most of the details for then, it would still be well to consider some examples here in order to add clarity to a statement of principles.

Ultrasound is an example of one current method of diagnosis. It is very widely used and almost everyone has probably heard of it. It enables the obstetrician to gain an abundance of information about the developing child and the condition of the mother. It is frequently used as a matter of course in prenatal examinations, in delivery and in various other procedures. It has been in general use for a number of years now. No one can prove beyond all doubt that it has no harmful side effects, but there are none of which anyone is aware. It seems both highly helpful and quite safe, with no apparent risk to mother or child.

Amniocentesis is another diagnostic method. It is invasive, which means that it can only be done by entering right into the body. The puncture of a needle through the abdominal wall, the uterus and right into the amniotic sac carries a degree of risk. There is a small possibility of miscarriage and the risk that the needle may touch and damage the unborn child — especially when it is done while the fetus is still extremely small. A great deal may be learned through it, but there are recognized risks. I think most people would see quite easily that, if you are truly concerned about the welfare of the unborn child, you should not do an invasive exam without a stronger reason than you would need for a routine exam by ultrasound.

If we are to come up with a good general principle based on both good medicine and good morals, then we might begin by saying this: Methods of diagnosis which have risks attached to them should not be used simply as a matter of course, but only when there are sufficiently serious reasons. It would follow, of course, that the more serious the risk, the more serious reason you would need in order to justify it. That is both good medical thinking and good moral thinking. Implied in this, of course, is the qualification that diagnostic procedures should be performed insofar as they are necessary. The necessity may include the fact that early diagnosis of certain conditions may make possible earlier and more effective treatment, if such be needed.

Included in our principles should also be the fact that procedures are not to be performed without the consent of the parents, since it is they who have the primary guardianship of the unborn child. The consent should be what is referred to as informed consent. This simply means that it is based on clear and honest explanation of what is to be done and why. This also is good practice morally, medically and even legally.

These items are all brought together in the *Instruction* in the form of one clear statement of principle: "Such diagnosis is permissible, with the consent of the parents after they have been adequately informed, if the methods employed safeguard the life and integrity of the embryo and the mother, without subjecting them to disproportionate risks."[41]

There still remains one additional and very important item to take into account. That is the question of motive. Diagnostic actions are seriously immoral when they are done in order to make possible a decision in favor of abortion. Sometimes diagnosis is performed to look for such things as Tay-Sachs disease or Sickle Cell Anemia or Downs Syndrome, with the intention of aborting the afflicted child. This would make the diagnosis an immoral act. "A diagnosis which shows the existence of a malformation or a hereditary illness must not be the equivalent of a death sentence."[42] This is bad moral practice, since we have no right to destroy innocent life. It is bad medical practice. In fact, it is insane medical practice, since only a madman sets out to fight disease by murdering his patients. It is, however, perfectly legal — to the lasting disgrace of our lawmakers and courts, and to those who do nothing to stop it.

Just as it is morally wrong to abort a child or to diagnose with intent to abort, so is it morally wrong for families, relatives or friends to counsel or encourage such procedures.

There are, of course, groups and programs which advocate the removal of defects by removing those who are defective. "Any directive or program of the civil and health authorities or of scientific organizations which in any way were to favor a link between parenatal diagnosis and

---

[41] *Instruction*, n. 31.

[42] *Instruction*, n. 31.

abortion, or which were to go so far as directly to induce expectant mothers to submit to prenatal diagnosis planned for the purpose of eliminating fetuses which are affected by malformations or which are carriers of hereditary illness, is to be condemned as a violation of the unborn child's right to life and as an abuse of the prior rights and duties of the spouses."[43]

Those who use diagnosis for this purpose take a potential good and distort it into an evil. Tell *them* where it hurts, and they'll get rid of *all* your pain.

---

[43] *Instruction*, n. 32.

# CHAPTER 15

## THE SEEING EAR AND OTHER MARVELS

For almost half of my life I was a teacher. In the beginning of those days, when everyone looked attentive and there were few questions, I used to congratulate myself on my clarity. It took me a while to learn to distinguish rapt attention from the steady gaze of self-hypnosis, and to realize that lack of questions sometimes meant that no one had any idea what I was talking about. Often enough it was as simple a matter as using words which were unfamiliar.

That is one of the reasons for this chapter. There are numerous procedures which can be used to examine a child while it is still in the uterus.[44] We are concerned, of course, with their moral implications. We cannot, however, make good moral judgments, unless we know the facts about how things work and what they are intended to do.

Diagnosis frequently involves the need to look into places that cannot ordinarily be seen. We are all familiar with X-rays, which pass through the body and form an image on a

---

[44] Some references for this and the following chapters come from: *The Merck Manual,* (hereafter referred to as *MM*) ed. 15, Merck Sharp and Dohme Research Laboratories, Rahway, N.J., 1987; Dr. Miriam Stoppard, *Everywoman's Medical Handbook* (hereafter referred to as *EMH*), Ballantine Books, N.Y. 1989.

photographic plate. With the aid of computers has come a much more sophisticated kind of X-ray called a CAT scan (CAT means Computer Assisted Tomography). There is another technique called MRI (Magnetic Resonance Imaging) which uses radio waves and a magnetic field. It is also possible to introduce various dyes or radioactive substances into the body, so that they can be traced for still further information.

Every one of these techniques has its own particular value in diagnosis, but during pregnancy every one of them also carries risks of harm or even death of the fetus. There are, however, still other possibilities.

*Sonography (ultrasound):* Sound waves can also penetrate tissue. They are reflected at various frequencies and those reflections (again with the aid of a computer) can be used to form an image (called a sonogram) on a video screen. The technique is totally painless. The skin is lubricated with a bit of oil so the small "microphone" can easily slide around, to emit and pick up the sound waves, which are neither felt nor heard (since they are beyond the range of our hearing). The technique works especially well on a rounded surface (such as the abdomen of a pregnant woman). The image also allows movement to be seen — even the beating heart of a fetus.

The sonogram can be of considerable help in both pregnancy and delivery. The process is non-invasive and allows the physician to be of more assistance to both mother and child. In making a moral judgement about the use of sonography, we should take into account not only how it works, but also why it is used.

It is of some use in certain problems with infertility. Since it is sensitive to even soft tissue, it can be used to view the stage of ripening follicles in order to know more precisely when ovulation will occur. It can also detect the presence of ovarian cysts, which are an impediment to fertility.

Once pregnancy begins, the fetus can be readily seen from the fourth or fifth week, so that both growth and position can be monitored.

Where there is threat of premature birth or when early delivery becomes necessary because of risk to either child or mother, some potential problems are offset by sonography. It makes it possible to get a visual image of fetal body size and head circumference. Both of these are important in assessing viability.

Should there be a need for amniocentesis or Chorionic Villus Sampling, ultrasound will be used in determining the precise position of the needle. It is used also to guide the instrument in the performance of intrauterine surgery or intrauterine transfusion.

Not only does sonography reveal the size and position of the fetus, but it also gives us that same information about the placenta (that portion of the fetal tissue which is attached to the uterine wall).

The position of the fetus can be quite critical as delivery approaches. So too is the position of the placenta. There is, for example, a condition known as placenta previa, in which the placenta is positioned in the uterus in such a way as to block the exit of the child in delivery. This not only impedes the ease of normal birth, it also can be the cause of severe bleeding. Ultrasound can alert a delivery team to take appropriate steps long before an emergency arises.

What can we say, at this point, about sonography (ultrasound)? There are clearly a number of perfectly good moral motives for using it. At present it seems quite safe and no undesirable side effects have been observed.[45]   In terms of moral judgment, sonography seems acceptable. Right now it's the best way to hear a picture.

*Amniocentesis*[46]:  The word means "a puncturing of the amnion."  The amnion is the innermost membrane of the sac of fluid in which the fetus is contained while within the uterus.  Amniocentesis is performed by passing a needle through the abdominal wall of the mother, through the wall of the uterus and into the amnion.  The needle is guided by means of sonography.  Through the needle a small amount of amniotic fluid is withdrawn.

Amniotic fluid is produced by the fetus and not by the mother.  Floating in it are some fetal cells which are used to prepare a tissue culture — which will take a few weeks. Since this is *fetal* tissue, it can be used to diagnose a variety of fetal conditions.

Amniocentesis can be done by the fifteenth or sixteenth week of pregnancy, since prior to then the fetus and amnion are simply too small and the needle could cause severe damage or even death.  Even at the later stage the process is quite delicate and can carry some risks for the fetus, causing miscarriage at a rate of about 1 per 200 (0.5%).

*Chorionic Villus Sampling* (CVS)[47]:  The chorion is the outermost layer of membrane around the embryo.  It has villi (hairlike structures) which embed in the wall of the

---

[45] It should be noted, however, that all possible serious side effects have not been disproven either -- and it took decades to see the harmful effects of x-ray.

[46] Cf. *MM*. pp.2156-2158; *EMH*, p. 81.

[47] Cf. *MM*, p. 2158; *EMH*, 124.

uterus. Both chorion and villi are part of the organs of the child rather than of the mother. CVS consists in inserting a needle (guided by sonography) through the mouth of the uterus or through the abdominal wall and through the wall of the uterus, to remove some of the chorionic cells. These can then be examined as a source for fetal diagnosis.

CVS is more risky than amniocentesis and anywhere from 2 to 6 miscarriages per 100 (2% to 6%) have been documented. There are insufficient data to make a judgement about harm to the fetus that goes on to term. CVS may be done in the eighth to tenth week of pregnancy. Since it offers more cells than can be obtained by amniocentesis, the results are available in a matter of days or hours rather than weeks.

I find it sad, however, to report that the main advantage of CVS over amniocentesis is described in the literature primarily in terms of making abortion decisions possible at an earlier date.

*Fetoscopy*[48]: This is a way of viewing the fetus directly. An incision is made in the mother's abdominal wall. A needle is inserted through the wall of the uterus and right into the amniotic sac. Contained within the needle are a light and a fiber optic lens. By this means the fetus can be examined visually in order to detect any visible abnormalities.

It is possible to perform fetoscopy beginning at about the fifteenth week of pregnancy. It is quite invasive and carries with it a high risk of miscarriage.

Apart from sonography, none of the procedures described above should be done simply as a matter of course. They

---

[48] Cf. *EMH*, p. 179.

are much too dangerous to the life of the fetus. When we make moral judgments about these or other procedures the element of risk must be taken into account. Such techniques should not be used unless the health or life of the fetus is already at some risk and the potential benefit to the child is at least as important as the risk being taken. Of course, they should not be done at all if they can be of no help to the fetus.

There is one point to be considered, and that is the purpose of the tests. If we are making a judgement about morality, then we must always consider the motive. The mere fact of a good motive does not justify an evil act. An evil motive, of course, is always morally wrong. If the tests described above are truly beneficial to the unborn child (for example, if they allow for some treatment to be started), and if they are necessary, then they *may* be morally justified — if they do not involve a risk which is more significant than the expected benefit. However, if such tests are being done with the intention of deciding to abort the child, then their use is morally wrong.

# CHAPTER 16

# LIES, DAMNED LIES AND STATISTICS

Pythagoras, simply in order to make life more difficult for all future generations of high school students, developed the theory that the square upon the hypotenuse of a right triangle is equal to the sum of the squares upon the other two sides.

What, you may ask, has that got to do with moral decisions or medical ethics? Nothing at all, so far as I know. But Pythagoras was enamored of numbers. He saw in them a magical quality and thought that they ruled the world and human lives as well. The fact is that, quaint as Pythagoras' ideas may seem to us, our own culture tends to do the same. Of course, we would never call that magic. We call it statistics. The national sport of baseball is immersed in them to point of absurdity. (Who was the only red-headed, left-handed pitcher with a wart on his nose to come within one run of a no-hitter on a cloudy day in Cleveland?) Those statistics are silly and inane, but completely harmless. Others may be far less amusing.

In the last chapter I spoke of amniocentesis. It is frequently used as a means of diagnosing possible genetic abnormalities in the developing child before its birth. All too often it is employed to make a decision on abortion. The decision as to whether to make use of amniocentesis is, to a large extent, based upon statistics.

104

A good example of this is the occurrence of the condition known as Down's Syndrome (also referred to as Trisomy 21 or Mongolism).[49] Children born with this condition have varying degrees of physical deformities and varying levels of mental retardation. It is a condition which can occur in any pregnancy, when the right genetic factors are present. The chances of having a Down's Syndrome child increase as the age of the mother increases. In fact, by the time a woman is 40 years of age, she is *50 times* more likely to have a Down's Syndrome child than is a woman of 20. That is an example of a statistic that sounds both shocking and frightening — but read on!

Many — doctors as well as others — interpret this as though it means that 50% of women over 40 are likely to have a Down's Syndrome child. Many are willing to kill a person who is so afflicted, and so they recommend abortion. They will advise that any woman who becomes pregnant over the age of 40, and perhaps even over 35, should undergo amniocentesis, with a view to possible abortion.

It is clear and obvious that the fact of physical affliction or mental retardation is not and never should be an excuse for killing a person. Hard as it is for many to admit, there is in our culture a dreadful bias against the handicapped. It is evident in an attitude which would hold that it is better to be dead. Or the bias may be founded in the even more frightening possibility that it is better to kill the handicapped than to care for them.

This attitude of rejection of the handicapped is made abundantly clear in one case in which the child had already

---

[49] Cf. *MM*, pp. 2145-2146; *EMH*, p. 160.

been born.   Infant Doe was born on April 9, 1982, in Bloomington, Indiana. He was born with tracheoesophogeal fistula, a condition which prevents swallowing. He could have been fed at first by intravenous injection, since neither food nor drink could be taken by mouth.   Corrective surgery, with a 90% success rate if done within 24 hours, was readily available at nearby Riley Children's Hospital. The obstetrician, however, offered the parents an alternative "treatment" of doing *nothing*.   The reason was that the infant had Down's Syndrome.

Both Doctor and parents argued that a Down's Syndrome child would never have a "minimally acceptable quality of life."  On June 10, Judge John Baker held a hearing at the hospital.  The obstetrician recommended keeping the baby in the hospital, but with no surgery, no food and no water. He based his statement on the fact that the surgery would cure the digestive problem, but would not cure the retardation.   Three other doctors testified and all recommended that Infant Doe be sent to Riley Children's Hospital for surgery.

On April 13 the county prosecutor brought a case to secure treatment for the child.   The same testimony was given. There was also another doctor who testified that no one could predict that the retardation would be serious, since Down's children may have an IQ ranging anywhere from 30 to normal range.  The obstetrician agreed, but still insisted on no treatment.  The court ruled that the child could be starved to death![50]

---

[50] Cf. Dennis J. Horan and Burke J. Balch, "Infant Doe and Baby Jane Doe: Medical Treatment of the Handicapped Newborn," in *Linacre Quarterly*, Vol. 52, 1985, 45-76; Brian V. Johnstone, "The Sanctity of Life, the Quality of Life and the New 'Baby Doe' Law," in *Linacre Quarterly*, Vol. 52, 1985. 258-270.

This bias against the handicapped is hard to overcome. The frightening statistics about the frequency of Down's Syndrome in older pregnant women adds to the fear. But what are the real numbers which lead to that fear?

Young mothers (those in their twenties) have a chance of 1 in 2000 of having a Down's Syndrome child. That is 0.05% (five one hundredths of one percent!), which means that their chances of having a child *without* Down's Syndrome are 99.95%.

By the time a woman reaches the age of 35, the chances go up to 1 in 200. That is a 0.5% (one-half of one percent!) chance of Down's — which is ten times higher than it is for the younger woman. Of course, that still means that there is a 99.5% chance of a baby *without* Down's.

At the ripe old age of 40, the woman's chances for a Down's baby will be 1 in 40, which is 2.5%. What then are her chances of having a child *without* Down's? A resounding 97.5%! The chance of a Down's child is indeed 50 times higher than it is for the woman who is twenty - but it is still less than 3%!

Yet there are women over 40 who become pregnant and abort their children through fear that they will be afflicted with Down's. Indeed, they are often enough encouraged to do so even without amniocentesis. The reason is that amniocentesis cannot be done until after the fifteenth week of pregnancy, and earlier abortions are easier to perform. Chorionic Villus Sampling may be done earlier — carrying with it, of course, a 6% chance of accidentally killing a child who has only a 2.5% chance of having Down's — and that is in the highest maternal age group.

Should every woman over the age of 35 have amniocentesis routinely done in order to see if Down's Syndrome is present. My response would be a clear, "NO!" The chances of a child with Down's is only 0.05%, and the chance of miscarriage from diagnosis is 0.5%. And even after Down's is diagnosed, abortion is still murder.

My point is not in any way to deny the sadness that will be, at least at first, experienced by those very few parents who do have a Down's Syndrome child. One point that I do want to make, however, is this: Numbers can convey a great deal of information, but they can be easily misread. There are also those who — out of ignorance, avarice, malice or stupidity — will misuse them for their own ends. Always check very carefully when you are being overwhelmed by statistics. They are not magic and they should not rule your life.

Am I giving good advice when I say that women over 35 should *not* have amniocentesis in order to diagnosis Down's. Or am I saying something stupid and irresponsible? At present it is very good advice indeed. I say "at present" because I do not discount the possibility that at some time in the future it may be possible to do something to correct Down's while the child is still in the womb. If that were the case, then it might be worth the risk. The intent in that instance would certainly be the welfare of the child. Right now that is not the case. The presence of Down's is sought simply so that the child can be killed, because it is imperfect. And let's be honest: If perfection is our criterion, then we are all in trouble — yea, even I, your humble servant!

What is Down's Syndrome, and why is there such fear of it? It is a genetic defect. The normal human cell has 46 chromosomes. These are the cell structures that contain the genes which determine all of our inherited characteristics. We receive 23 chromosomes from our mothers and 23 from our fathers. These have been grouped and numbered by

108

scientists and can be observed. The Down's Syndrome child characteristically (95% of the time) has 47 chromosomes instead of the usual 46. There is an extra chromosome in group 21.

This is what is detected in the cells cultured from amniocentesis. It is why the Syndrome is called Trisomy 21, which simply means that there are three chromosomes in group 21 rather than the normal two. It is referred to as Mongolism because of certain physical characteristics (shape of nose, eyes, etc.).

Not very long ago it was assumed that the Down's Syndrome child was always severely retarded and was best institutionalized for life. That, of course, was a self-fulfilling prophecy. Any child put into an institution, taught nothing, removed from family, and given little environmental stimulation will not fail to match our lowest expectations. In those circumstances even a normal child would probably show signs of serious retardation.

What are the facts? There are some physical defects which may be life threatening. About one-third of these children may have heart problems and could die at an early age. The rest live into adulthood, but age more quickly and have a life expectancy of 40 to 60 years.

The severity of retardation varies. The average IQ is about 50 (50 to 70 is considered *mild* retardation). This means, of course, that some are over 50 and some below. It also means that the former assumption of inevitable severe retardation is totally inaccurate. Yet there are still many — including some doctors — who continue to propagate this error.

Given early stimulation and attention, and with continued education, Down's Syndrome children can cope quite well. Some may continue to need a good bit of help, while others can become capable of holding responsible jobs. But there is something even more important. The common qualities I have *personally* observed in Down's Syndrome children are gentleness, trust and a beautiful desire to love and be loved.

What is really stupid and irresponsible? Is it the desire to see these children have a chance to live? Or is it the compulsion to kill them before they can draw their first breath?

# CHAPTER 17

## ARE WE WINNING THE WAR?

Do you recall, not so many years ago, when one of our political slogans was the "War on Poverty"? It is hard to say what stage we have reached in that war. Perhaps, indeed, the poor we shall always have with us... at least so long as we hold on so tightly to our selfishness.

In any case, would you consider it a benefit to humanity and to human dignity, if you were told that the war was being won because we had succeeded at last in killing off the last poor person? Would you consider it moral — or even sane — if you were told that you ought to search out and kill a poor person for the benefit of society?

What about the war on hereditary diseases? Should it be fought by seeking out and killing those who are its victims? Or should we be looking for a better way to counteract the disease itself?

There are two hereditary diseases which have been widely publicized. These are Tay-Sachs disease and Sickle Cell Anemia. Another, which is probably less well known, is Thalassemia. All three have been addressed in similar ways. One method is to screen carriers and encourage them not to have children. This approach includes the use of sterilization or birth control. Another method is to use amniocentesis to determine the presence of the disease in unborn children and then abort them.

All three of these conditions are hereditary, all are connected with particular ethnic or racial groups. All three are or can be quite serious, even fatal.

Tay-Sachs disease is most common among those who are of Eastern European Jewish origin, although perhaps only about 4% of that group carry the genes connected with this affliction.[51] It is 100 times more rare in other groups. The carriers do not themselves have the disease, but they do have the genes which lead to it. When it is inherited, its effects occur very early in life. There is a progressively retarded development of the victim. An enzyme deficiency results in damage to the brain. This results in dementia, paralysis and blindness. Death will occur by the age of three or four.

Sickle Cell Anemia is found almost always in those of African origin.[52] It, too, is a serious disease. Its name comes from the fact that red blood cells, which should be circular disks in shape, are instead sickle shaped. As the name of the disease indicates, its victims suffer from anemia. There are stages in which the bone marrow slows down in its production of red blood cells. There may be fever, vomiting and abdominal pain, pain in the back and joints. There may be poor body development and changes in bone structure visible on X-ray. There is no cure, but some treatment can be given for the symptoms. Lifespan has increased to more than 40 years, and death may finally come from such causes as infection, kidney failure or blockage of blood vessels in some vital area.

---

[51] Cf. *MM*, pp. 1013, 2140, 2158-2159.

[52] Cf. *MM*, pp. 1120-1121, 2159.

112

Thalassemia also affects certain ethnic groups.[53] One type is found among those of Mediterranean origin. There is another which is found among Orientals. Some forms are mild and may require no treatment. Others are far more severe. Symptoms can be quite serious and may include anemia, jaundice, impairment of growth, liver disease and even heart failure. Life expectancy varies in the different forms. In some it is normal, in others it may be as low as the early teens.

None of these diseases is really common. However, my purpose in describing them is not to say that we are all in danger of contracting them. On the other hand, I want to make it clear that, although rare, they are quite severe. There is no doubt that those who suffer from them deserve a great deal of concern and compassion.

On the other hand, it should be clearly stated that killing those who have these diseases is murder and cannot be justified out of the desire to rid humanity of an affliction or some totally fictitious sort of compassion. We should address the diseases and search for a cure, but it is morally wrong and dehumanizing to wipe out the afflicted. At the present stage of medicine, diagnosis of these conditions by amniocentesis serves no morally good purpose. No cure is offered and the only result is the death of one more casualty in a twisted sort of war on disease.

---

[53] Cf. *MM*, pp. 1122-1124, 2159.

# CHAPTER 18

## BACK IN THE SADDLE AGAIN

Early in the American Civil War it became clear that all the best generals seemed to have gone South.  The Union army lacked leadership and one general replaced another with alarming alacrity.  In June of 1862, Lincoln appointed General John Pope to command of the army around Washington — a choice which proved unhappy when he marched boldly off into the disaster of the second battle of Bull Run.

Pope set out in a flurry, as if to make up for his predecessor's chronic inactivity.  The story (perhaps apocryphal) is told that he sent a report to the president signed, rather dramatically, "from my headquarters in the saddle." Lincoln's comment was along the lines of, "And now we have a general whose headquarters are where his hindquarters ought to be."

In some ways our reaction to new scientific achievements is as misplaced as was the general's burst of enthusiasm. We leap unthinkingly into new areas and end up getting everything backwards.

In the last few chapters I looked at a number of conditions which can be diagnosed in the uterus by means of amniocentesis. For none of them do we have a cure.  In each instance, once the diagnosis is made, there is still no treatment that can be offered.

Many, however, like that same general, seem to put their headquarters where their hindquarters ought to be. Seeing a disease, and having no cure, they decide simply to forge ahead and banish the disease by killing the person who has it.

This sort of conduct we must totally reject. This does not mean that we must necessarily denounce amniocentesis as immoral, although in the cases mentioned thus far it is, since its *purpose* is immoral in each instance. It does, however, have some good and proper uses, and may have even more in the future.

It may well happen that science will be able to develop techniques to treat or even to cure some of the genetic disorders that I have spoken of earlier. It may even become possible to do so while the child is still in the womb. Amniocentesis will then be a valuable and life saving tool, and its relatively small risks will be far outweighed by its potential benefit to the unborn child. At the present time its use as a means of helping people to decide for abortion is a dreadful misuse of a potential good.

We should, however, make a distinction. Amniocentesis becomes possible in the *second trimester*. The fact is, though, that at our present state of knowledge and ability, it serves no useful purpose at that stage. It can determine defects, but there is nothing that can be done about them. It offers no help to the infant. It can also discover the sex of the child, but that knowledge likewise is of no use — except to those who wish to abort a child of the "wrong" sex. (This is an example of the schizophrenic nature of the abortionist. Shout out the slogans about the evils of sexism and then proclaim the right to a sexism that is not only discriminatory but homicidal.)

Use of amniocentesis in the *third trimester* may be quite different. In those last three months of pregnancy it has, even now, some quite legitimate and even life saving uses. One of those functions, in the case of a condition called erythroblastosis fetalis, is a perfect example not only of a good use, but also of what happens when medicine is willing to look past abortion and seek a real solution to a problem.[54]

Erythroblastosis fetalis (also called Rhesus incompatibility) is a blood problem which can be serious and even life threatening. It comes about under specific conditions and happens only to certain couples.

When a mother has Rh-negative blood and the father has Rh-positive, the child may inherit either one. If the child has Rh-negative, the same as the mother, there is no problem. Even if the child has Rh-positive, there still may be no problem — unless a certain series of events takes place.

If a person with Rh-negative blood receives a transfusion of Rh-positive, the body recognizes this blood as foreign and tries to protect itself against it. It forms anti-bodies to fight off the invasion. Even after the threat is over, the anti-bodies remain. This is, in fact, similar to what happens in a vaccination. The body forms anti-bodies capable of fighting off that same infection, should it ever return.

Under normal conditions there is no mixing of blood between mother and child. The two systems are in close proximity through the placenta. Nourishment and waste can be passed back and forth, but the blood cells do not make

---

[54] Cf. *MM*, pp. 1766-1768, 1875-1877; *EMH*, p. 300.

direct contact. It is possible, however, for anti-bodies to pass back and forth. This is when the problem begins.

Anti-bodies from the mother will see Rh-positive blood cells as an enemy to be destroyed. When they enter the blood of the Rh-positive baby, they begin attacking the red blood cells (erythrocytes). The result is anemia in the child, and its system fights back by producing more red cells in its bone marrow. If it can't keep up with the attack, it will begin sending immature red blood cells (erythroblasts) into the blood stream. The anemia may even become severe enough to kill the unborn child.

How does the mother become sensitized and begin producing these anti-bodies? I already mentioned one way — transfusion. It can also occur if there is some accident in the placenta and the blood of mother and child are allowed to mix. It may easily happen at the time of delivery, when the placenta pulls away from the uterine wall and bleeding occurs. This may lead to problems in future pregnancies.

Usually there is no problem with the first child, provided that the mother has not previously had a transfusion of Rh-positive blood. Once the condition begins, however, each succeeding pregnancy may have more and more serious problems. In fact, there was a time when, by the third or fourth child, the chances were relatively high that it would die before birth. This is no longer the case, as I shall explain.

As recently as fifteen or twenty years ago, the medical literature often recommended performing an abortion when blood tests of the mother showed a rise in antibodies. The literature also recommended contraceptive sterilization to prevent future problems. It was the same "easy way out" that we find recommended so often in other instances and

117

is no therapy at all, since it merely kills the one who is ill, or destroys the power to procreate. A more honest therapeutic approach has since been developed, an approach which seeks to save life and not to destroy it.

Some of the possibilities of therapy depend upon the use of amniocentesis. In this case its use is morally justified. There is, of course, some risk from the procedure itself, but that risk is lessened in the third trimester, and the amniocentesis is being done to benefit the unborn child and, perhaps, to save its life. The smaller risk of the technique is worth taking in order to overcome the greater risk of disease. In addition, the motive is morally good. Let me explain what amniocentesis does in this instance.

As the anti-bodies from the mother cause breakdown of the baby's red blood cells, they produce a red pigment called bilirubin. This is, for the most part, carried off as waste transfer through the placenta. Some of it, however, will also be found in the amniotic fluid. The rise in this, as well as a rise in anti-bodies in the mother's blood, are a sign of problems.

If the mother's anti-bodies rise too high, then it is time to make use of amniocentesis in order to examine the bilirubin level in the amniotic fluid. This would usually begin at about the twenty-sixth to twenty-eighth week of pregnancy. It will probably be repeated about every two weeks. If the levels of bilirubin remain in an acceptable range, nothing more need be done. Monitoring will continue and pregnancy can go on to term.

If the levels of bilirubin continue to rise, it may be necessary to perform a blood transfusion while the child is still in the uterus. This is done by use of amniocentesis guided by ultrasound. This may be repeated at intervals until the child is more safely viable. At that time labor may be induced.

Even after birth, there may be more which needs to be done. The bilirubin, which was being carried off through the placenta, may now begin to rise in the child. If allowed to continue, this could result in brain damage leading to death or to other complications, such as hearing problems or mental retardation. This, however, can also be prevented. The doctor delivering the baby will be prepared to do an exchange blood transfusion, which will clear the child's blood and bring it back to normal.

In other words, there are now methods of diagnosis and treatment which will head off and correct a situation which at one time would probably have been fatal. These methods, of course, will demand more than the usual care and will probably be done in specially equipped hospitals or medical centers.

It is helpful also to know that it is often possible to prevent this problem from occurring at all, provided that the mother has not previously received a transfusion of Rh-positive blood. Whenever she gives birth to a child who is Rh-positive she can receive injections of gamma-globulin to prevent the continued development of anti-bodies. Thus, even if the child's blood has gotten into her blood stream at the time of birth, its bad effects are prevented.

It should be pointed out also that the occurrence of this condition depends on having a husband who is Rh-positive, a wife who is Rh-negative and a child who is Rh-positive. Only about 13% of all marriages are between a man who is Rh-positive and a woman who is Rh-negative. Out of *those* marriages, only about 4% (i.e., 0.5% of *all* marriages) will have a problem. In other words, the condition is relatively rare.

The real point I want to make is this: When medical science is not seduced by abortion as a solution, it is capable of finding some truly amazing ways of saving life. Once we stop sitting on our heads and begin, instead, to think, the real potential for good seems endless.

## CHAPTER 19
## REINVENTING THE WHEEL

We come into the world as innocent babes. Innocent morally and every other way — innocent of language, innocent of knowledge, innocent even of potty training. How hard life would be if we had to start from scratch. No speech until we reinvent language; no learning until we reinvent books and all the knowledge needed to fill them; no potty training until we reinvent plumbing. Life would be a long, hard (and somewhat unsanitary) process.

The good news is that every generation inherits the discoveries and memories of earlier generations and can begin life from there. That is one of the blessings of tradition, which is simply the handing on of all that has gone before us. This is also true in the area of morality. We are not forced to start without a clue about right or wrong and try to work it all out on our own — although we sometimes seem to want to do just that. The tradition of the Church is a gold mine of information about morality, yet it is all too often set aside as people try to figure out what they ought to do.

In this chapter I would like to complete our consideration of intrauterine diagnosis and treatment. I will present still one more example of a good and proper use for amniocentesis. This will be followed by an example of an effort to make a decision between right and wrong. It is a recounting of a legal decision involving the use of amniocentesis that I am about to give. Finally, I will summarize the basic principles which ought to be taken into account in any such decision. Let me begin with this one more use of amniocentesis.

The unborn child reaches a point at which it becomes possible for it to live outside the uterus. That is to say, it has become viable.[55] That point comes long before the end of the ninth month of pregnancy. Between then and the end of the ninth month, the child grows larger, stronger and far better suited for survival. Yet there are situations in which early delivery is unavoidable. The mother may simply go into labor long before the date when the baby is due. It may also happen that some medical crisis makes it necessary to deliver the baby at an early date, and labor is therefore purposely induced. The child born early will have a harder time surviving. It has need of some special care if it is going to live. Modern medicine has evolved techniques which have greatly increased the survival rate at dates much earlier than would once have been possible.

When pregnancy reaches the twenty-third or twenty-fourth week, the child is viable — with some considerable and very special help. The more premature the infant, the more problems there may be. Not so very long ago a child born before the twenty-sixth week would probably have died. New techniques have made a vast difference. When you consider how much growth and maturity takes place in each week of pregnancy — especially during the first six months — the change in time of viability has been significant indeed.

---

[55] Cf. *MM*, pp. 1852-1871.

Earlier delivery means difficulties in a variety of areas. The central nervous system continues to develop up to and even after the time of birth. A child born more than six weeks before term (term is considered to be the fortieth week and a baby born before the thirty-seventh week is considered premature) may therefore have some problems with reflexes of sucking and may need to be fed intravenously or by means of a stomach tube.

The premature infant has a less well developed gastrointestinal tract. In addition to a problem with sucking and swallowing, it also has a small stomach. This problem can be alleviated by using a tube to feed the infant human milk or special formulas. There may also be problems due to immature kidneys or high bilirubin levels. These can also be aided by ordinary and rather readily available procedures. (Of course, I do not mean that all procedures are available in all hospitals. In this country, however, there are enough hospitals which supply this sort of care, so that it is possible to deliver in one of them or to take the newborn there shortly after birth.)

There is one area, however, in which little assistance can be given at the present time. This is why the present limit on viability is between the twenty-third and twenty-fourth weeks. The area to which I refer is that of lung maturity.[56] While the fetus is in the uterus, oxygen and carbon dioxide are passed between mother and child through the placenta. The lungs of the infant are filled, not with air, but with amniotic fluid. The fetus does have respiratory movements even in the uterus, but what is "breathed" in and out is fluid. In fact, before the twenty-third week of pregnancy,

---

[56] Cf. *MM*, pp. 1799-1801.

the inner surface of the lungs is not sufficiently developed to allow gases (oxygen and carbon dioxide) to pass to or from the blood system. Breathing air is, therefore, impossible.[57]

If it becomes necessary for the welfare of child and mother to induce labor at a very early stage, one serious concern will be whether the lungs are sufficiently developed. Sonograms, of course, can show the size of the infant and this may sometimes be sufficient to ensure that it has reached an age of at least twenty-four weeks — meaning that it is just at the stage when its lungs should be developed enough for viability.

Yet there are cases in which the size of the fetus may not be enough indication to guarantee lung maturity. When the exact week of pregnancy is not known (and it is not unusual for estimates to be off by as much as four weeks), a fetus may happen to be large for its age and yet have immature lungs. In fact, this is often the case when the mother suffers from diabetes mellitus. Her child will often tend to be larger than usual for its actual age. Mere size, however, does not prove lung maturity.

How, then, is it possible to tell before delivery if the lungs are sufficiently mature? The solution is amniocentesis. As I mentioned earlier, the unborn child "breathes" amniotic fluid. As the lungs come to maturity they produce

---

[57] There is presently no way to supply for a serious deficiency in lung maturity. However, on August 29, 1989, there appeared in *The New York Times* (p. C5) an article by Gina Kolata describing the action of a team of doctors at Temple University in Philadelphia. In an effort to save a premature infant they put an oxygen carrying liquid into her lungs. The child still died 19 hours later, but it is a hint of future possibilities. The article also mentioned that similar procedures used in experiments on animals have kept alive some that would have been equivalent to a twenty-week human fetus.

a substance called a surfactant. Particles of this are exhaled into the amniotic fluid and can be detected by amniocentesis. This allows for a morally good use of the procedure in order to help ensure the survival of the unborn.

Since we are looking at this particular use of amniocentesis, it seems appropriate also at this point to call attention to a recent event in which this was one of the points at issue.

On Wednesday, April 26, 1989, the Supreme Court of the United states heard the case of *Webster v. Reproductive Health Services*. The case had arisen from a Missouri law intended to place some limits on abortion and abortion funding.[58]

The State of Missouri was attempting by law to assert its right to protect human life in the womb. Even the wrong and utterly regrettable *Roe v. Wade* decision of 1973 had recognized the rights of the states to set some limit. Chief Justice Rehnquist, in the decision on the Missouri law, referred back to what had been said in *Roe v. Wade*. He wrote: "In *Roe v. Wade*, the court recognized that the state has 'important and legitimate' interest in protecting maternal health and in the potentiality of human life... During the second trimester, the state 'may, if it chooses, regulate the abortion procedure in ways that are reasonably related to maternal health'... After viability, when the state's interest in potential human life was held to be compelling, the state 'may, if it chooses, regulate, and even proscribe [i.e., forbid], abortion except where it is necessary, in

---

[58] Quotations from the laws involved and from the decision are taken from the opinions of the Justices as reprinted in *Origins, CNS Documentary Service*, July 13, 1989, Vol. 19: No. 9, pp. 129-151.

appropriate medical judgment, for the preservation of the life or health of the mother.'"

The Missouri statute being challenged in 1989 had said: "No abortion of a viable unborn child shall be performed unless necessary to preserve the life or health of the woman." It is saying that a child capable of living outside the womb should not be murdered as a matter of "choice." That is surely a very modest objective in the effort to protect human life, especially since there should *never* be a reason to kill such a child, since it can be delivered instead! That was also *one* clear and obvious flaw in *Roe v. Wade.*

Since the Missouri law was quite serious about protecting the viable child, it also took steps to make sure that viability would be properly determined. It stated: "Before a physician performs an abortion on a woman he has reason to believe is carrying an unborn child of 20 or more weeks gestational age, the physician shall first determine if the unborn child is viable by using and exercising that degree of care, skill and proficiency commonly exercised by the ordinarily skillful, careful and prudent physician engaged in similar practice under the same or similar conditions. In making this determination of viability, the physician shall perform or cause to be performed such medical examination and tests as are necessary to make a finding of the gestational age, weight and lung maturity of the unborn child and shall enter such findings and determination of viability in the medical record of the mother."

The law seems simple enough. The ordinary tests are required and results are to be made a matter of record. The law was signed into effect by the governor of Missouri in June of 1986. By December of the same year it was in court. The District Court stopped enforcement of the law

126

and it was struck down by the Eighth Circuit Court of Appeals in 1988. In reference to the tests for viability it said that they were an unconstitutional intrusion on a matter of medical skill and judgment. The same court said that tests for fetal weight at 20 weeks are inaccurate and would add $125 to $250 to the cost of an abortion. It was also of the opinion that "amniocentesis, the only method available to determine lung maturity, is contrary to accepted medical practice until 28-30 weeks of gestation, expensive and imposes significant health risks for both the pregnant woman and the fetus."

The Circuit Court seems to have been hunting for reasons to overturn the law — reasons to avoid further inconvenience to those who were already concerned enough about their own convenience to kill for it. The Court seemed somewhat misinformed as well. They see the tests for viability as an intrusion. The tests, of course, are no more than any doctor *should* do if there is a question of viability. Indeed, the law does not even require all of the tests all of the time; it requires only those needed to resolve the issue when there is reason for doubt. What did the Circuit Court prefer? A random guess? However, I suppose that if they did not want to save the lives at least of viable infants, then it didn't much matter to them if there were any tests at all.

The Circuit Court was missing the point or was really misinformed when it said that tests for fetal weight at 20 weeks are inaccurate and therefore not needed — besides they add extra expense to abortion. Even tests which are not totally accurate are accurate enough to indicate whether the baby is at an age of 20 rather than 24 weeks — and that, as I shall explain below, is one of the issues here. Furthermore, they simply separate the utility of amniocentesis from the other tests and fail to see the intent of the whole process. If the child is clearly large enough to be

127

viable, then there is no need for amniocentesis. If the size is on the edge between viability and non-viability, then there could be real doubt about lung maturity. That could be resolved by amniocentesis.

It is one more sign of misinformation when they speak of accepted medical practice as using amniocentesis only after 28-30 weeks of pregnancy. Doctors interested in saving a child would probably (apart from emergency delivery) use it only then. Those who favor abortion are not at all hesitant to use it at 15-16 weeks in order to track down and kill whomever they consider defective — explaining all the while how safe it is.

They then take leave of their senses completely and argue that amniocentesis poses "significant health risks for both the pregnant woman and the fetus." In terms of risk to the mother, amniocentesis is no problem at all compared to the risk she runs by having an abortion. The real risk is to the infant. Remember, however, that the law is dealing with all of this in the context of someone who is seeking an abortion. With no apology at all to the Court, I would ask one question: Would I be far wrong if I said that only an idiot would advocate killing a child without tests, on the ground that the tests would be hazardous to its health?

One more point about the law: It said that viability must be tested at 20 weeks. Of course, a fetus is not viable until almost 24 weeks. Why, then, the early test? Two reasons, I would say. The first is that mistakes of four weeks are not at all uncommon without testing. The second is that, in the instance envisioned by the legislators, the doctor doing the testing is most likely to be your local, friendly abortionist. He is in the habit of lying to women about their unborn children in any case. The law at least requires him to take one honest look at reality, and to keep a record of it.

Personally, I wouldn't put much faith even in their records, but it is at least an attempt to make them honest. Let us not forget, however, that the doctor in question also has a monetary interest in performing the abortion, so a legal requirement is also an effort to place some checks on greed.

Who do you suppose were the witnesses who told the Court of Appeals about the unfair price hike for testing and the risks of amniocentesis at 20 weeks? It was brought to them, I am sure, by those same wonderful folks who brought us abortion on demand and the total safety of amniocentesis when it can be used to promote abortion. People who don't mind killing probably don't mind lying either.

The approach taken by the court has one basic and fatal flaw. It fails to accept the *fact* that the unborn child is a human being and, therefore, a person. I speak of this as a fact rather than a theory because, as I have shown earlier, it is based on perfectly clear and valid inference from all the provable facts of science.

When all of the evidence is examined, we find that we have *no* reason to say that the unborn child is not a person. Once we accept the fact of the humanity of the fetus, then we *must* treat it with all the respect due to any person — and that includes the right to live. This is the point at which legality and morality come into conflict in our own age on the question of abortion. The courts have continued to take a one-sided view of the woman's rights, while refusing to examine or acknowledge the scientific facts. This leaves them in the position of constantly trying to reinvent the wheel. They are forced to act on a purely pragmatic base, because the objective foundation is simply set aside. Once the fact of humanity is accepted, then there is a perfectly valid legal tradition of respect for persons which makes life-saving decisions prevail over death-dealing ones.

I have presented a number of examples of diagnosis and therapy on the unborn, and I have offered conclusions on the morality of decisions we must make in regard to them. Those conclusions were not random, they were not pragmatic, they were not guesses. They began with the acceptance of the fact that the unborn child is a human person. This was followed by the application of simple, traditional principles that would serve the courts as easily as they serve moral theology. The principles are clear and simple and founded in normal common sense. The medical procedures are complex and so we must examine them very carefully in order to know what they do and how they do it. Once we understand the procedures, however, the principles are easy to use.

The basic principles for diagnosis and therapy on the unborn are simple enough. (1) The procedure must be beneficial (healing, therapeutic) for the unborn child. (2) It must respect and seek to preserve the life of the child. (3) It must seek to preserve the integrity (completeness) of the child. (4) It must not involve risks that are out of proportion to the good that can be accomplished for the child. (5) It must seek the improvement of the child's health and its survival. In view of present attitudes in society, I have emphasized the welfare of the child. It is obvious also that procedures intended to benefit the child should not be such as to cause harm to the mother either.

When you try to make a moral judgement about a procedure, learn all that you can about it and then ask how it fits in with each of these principles. If you are not sure, then consult with someone who can help you. Truly good

130

medical practice will go along completely with every one of those principles.

There is still one more factor to be taken into account. Nothing should be done without the free and informed consent of the parents. This means that parents have the right to full information about what is going to be done, why, its results and its chances of success. It is only on this basis that they will have the opportunity to make a decision that is good both medically and morally. In both areas we should take advantage of all the wisdom that has preceded us and we will have no need to reinvent the wheel.

# CHAPTER 20

## DOCTOR FRANKENSTEIN, I PRESUME

In 1931 *Frankenstein* came to the screen. Clive Colin was the misguided doctor who tried to play God and create human life. Boris Karloff made his debut as the monster. Who among us has not thrilled at least once to the sight of his awkward movements? We can all picture that flat head, the electrodes protruding from the neck and the thoroughly unstylish wedgies — upon which he clomped his way to stardom.

The movie was, of course, a success and is now considered a classic. It was entertainment, but it also held out to us that little chill of horror that makes the adrenalin flow — even though we know full well that the fright is only fictional. Yet the movie had a point to make as well. Man is *not* God and his efforts to make himself the Creator and Lord of life are doomed to distortion and disaster.

Still, it was just a movie. No one would really try to make a living man out of bits and pieces of dead bodies. And certainly no one would ever experiment on living human beings and then discard them. Well, maybe no one would have done it in 1931, but I wouldn't bet on it now.

In fact, only ten years after the movie, the Nazis were planning a "master race," and were cutting up the living bodies of people whom they had first declared non-human and therefore available for experiment. Today the original Nazis are gone, but their successors are ready and willing to pick up where they left off. The new madmen have classified the unborn as non-human and they are now busily cutting up small bodies, both living and dead, for their "noble" experiments.

There is no doubt at all that science — including medical science — is advanced by experiment. There is no doubt that experimentation has led frequently to results which have bettered or even saved human life. The principles enunciated or presupposed in the *Instruction on Procreation* are certainly not opposed to the need of science and medicine for deeper, knowledge. Nor are they opposed to the need for research and experiment. What the document does constantly take into account, however, is that deeper knowledge of human beings must never cease to be viewed as deeper knowledge of *persons*. The scientific tendency to tunnel vision[59] should never reduce the scientist to seeing the human being only as a collection of parts to be analyzed. Research or experiment on living human beings must always keep before it the awareness that we are dealing with *persons* and not simply with tissue.

In an experiment on a material object (e.g., stress tests on steel components for bridge construction), the object may be broken or destroyed in the process. Experiments on animals should be done with care to minimize pain or suffering — not because animals are persons, but because we (the experimenters) are. Animal experiment may result in injury or death; but the results, in terms of benefit to persons, may be used as moral justification to warrant the loss. This is not the case when the object of experiment is a human being. Human beings should not be broken or

---

[59] Cf. supra, Chapter 2.

destroyed, nor should they be wilfully subjected to injury or death.

The researcher must *never* lose sight of the fact that he is dealing with a person. This is most especially the case in respect to the unborn, who have no way to protect or safeguard themselves, but must depend totally on us. The norms of moral theology are quite clear in this area, and we shall look at them shortly. Let us begin, however, by looking at just what is meant by "research" and "experimentation." In the minds of many, the two words may seem practically identical. In the *Instruction*, however, they are used more carefully and I will try to be equally careful in the way in which I use them here.

*Research* refers to a systematic process of observation. It is primarily a matter of looking, keeping records and learning from this information. It would be neither painful nor harmful and certainly not fatal. It should be non-invasive. Of course, the means of observation are important. For example, examining the workings of someone's mind by watching his actions is far different from doing it by opening up his head. In the case of a fetus, the use of X-ray as a means of observation could be quite harmful, while sonographic examination seems not to be.

*Experiment* is more than observation. It involves not only research (looking) but active intervention (doing something). Experiment on a human being (at any stage of life, from zygote to adult) *involves doing something to a person.* In medicine this could involve the performance of surgical procedures or the use of drugs or new technologies. the purpose is to verify some result or effect which is not yet known or not yet understood.

But, you may ask, why take up this question of fetal research or experiment at any great length? It would seem

134

that any dangerous procedure performed on a fetus would be done only as a last ditch effort to save its life, and surely no one would object seriously to that. It is true that an emergency of that sort could justify a great deal of heroic effort. (In fact, we will in a later chapter offer some principles in this regard.) The fact is, however, that our laws have little or no regard for the unborn and they have become subject to the worst sort of cruel experimentation.

One book that I would recommend for your reading in this area is *Beyond Abortion: A Chronicle of Fetal Experimentation*, by Suzanne M. Rini.[60] If the book does nothing else, it will at least assure you that Dr. Frankenstein is not dead. Allow me to give you some examples of what she says — although I will omit the names of persons involved since I don't wish to take all the space which would be required for all the supporting documentation (all of which you will find in Rini's book).

There are examples not only of the use of fetuses for experiment, but also of the lowest forms of crass commercialism. One Washington, D.C., hospital, for example, in 1976 was found not only to have charged women to perform abortions on them, but had then sold their dead children for use in experiments. The sales resulted in an income of some $88,000! They explained, however, that is was all in a good cause. The money was used to send doctors to conventions and to purchase cookies and soft drinks for visiting professors.

In 1982 in California a container company set out to repossess one of its containers which was being used by a

---

[60] Cf. Suzanne M. Rini, *Beyond Abortion: A Chronicle of Fetal Experimentation*, Magnificat Press, 1988.

pathologist. Workers were horrified to discover that it was full of fetuses stacked in jars and cartons. In fact, there were more than 16,000 of them, some as far developed as five months. (That, of course, is frightful to contemplate, but it is still only one per-cent of a single year's abortion in the United States alone.) The bodies had come from doctors and clinics in California and Missouri.

The case was brought to the attention of the district attorney and he tried to take legal steps to have them buried. His efforts were blocked by a law suit brought by the ACLU on behalf of a women's health center. Treating them as human bodies might set the dangerous legal precedent of treating fetuses themselves as human! Years later the stacked bodies were still in their original containers, as the court case dragged on.

In incidents in Canada in the early and mid-1970's more than 50 fetuses were delivered alive by hysterotomy. (Hysterotomy is another one of those more "antiseptic" words the abortionists love to use. It is, in fact, a Caesarean section, but calling it that would make it too evident that the intent was to deliver and then murder these children.) The fetuses ranged from ten to twenty-five weeks gestational age (the latter, of course, viable). Upon delivery they were cut open — while alive — and had their adrenal glands and sex organs removed for experiment. This case finally resulted in criminal charges against the participants.

Have you ever wondered what happens to the children who are murdered at your local abortion mills? If you are interested in a possible pro-life project, try stirring up the local media people to do some investigative reporting. Whatever the results, they will certainly be interesting.

What are the "noble" experiments for which these living and dead children are so essential? We can look at that in

136

the next chapter. For right now I just wanted you to know that Dr. Frankenstein is alive and well — and prospering right here in our own country.

# CHAPTER 21

# SCIENTIFIC CYCLOPES

"How many learned men are working at the forge of science — laborious, ardent, tireless Cyclopes, but one-eyed!"[61] The Cyclopes, those fearsome creatures of Greek mythology. They were the favorites of Zeus, his artisans who forged the thunderbolts which were his weapons. He put them in a land where they had all they needed. But they were also creatures without law and subject to no courts of justice.[62] Talent, ability, power — and chaos. Their name means "wheel-eyed," for each had only one eye, as big as a cartwheel, in the middle of his forehead. Perhaps this accounts for their fierce, chaotic nature. It takes two eyes to have depth perception, and depth perception is essential if we are to have perspective and be able to see the proper relation between one thing and another.

Experimentation on fetuses is a perfect example of this one-eyed, flat, dimensionless vision of the scientific Cyclopes. There are those who perform the most atrocious experiments, yet try to make their work seem noble. They describe their goals in terms of the good that will be

---

[61] Joseph Joubert, *Pensées*, 1842.

[62] Cf. Edith Hamilton, *Mythology*, Mentor Books, 1963, pp. 65,81-82, 168, 222, 280.

achieved for "humanity," while they routinely tear apart living human beings. Their flat vision fixes its focus on an abstraction, all the while ignoring real, living persons. They may, indeed, gain some knowledge from what they do, but their purposes are by no means so noble as they would have us believe. In 1981 an internationally known drug company was reported to have made arrangements with an Arizona abortion clinic to take part in an experiment.[63] Free abortions were provided for 14 women who agreed to cooperate. All of them, while pregnant, were given an experimental drug intended for use in the treatment of hypertension. Each day, during the course of medication, blood was taken from the women and amniotic fluid was drawn from their wombs for examination.

The drawing of the amniotic fluid is, of course, always to some degree risky to the fetus. The medicine taken by the women may also have been harmful. In fact, the intent of the procedure was to see what effect it would have. These factors alone would be enough to make the whole procedure wrong, since they indicate a callous risk to fetal life in order to acquire knowledge and with no benefit whatsoever to the fetus.

What happened next, however, was utterly and totally wrong. All 14 of the women were given prostaglandins to induce abortions and their children were then delivered — in order to be killed and have their bodies examined for effects of the drug. The report said that the hospital received $10,000 — a sizeable increase over the $2800 to $3200 that they might have expected as their usual abortion fee if the women had paid. Each of the women, it would

---

[63] For details, cf. Suzanne M. Rini, *op. cit.*, p. 37. I also wrote to the drug company asking for information on this, but I never received an answer.

seem, got nothing but the possible side effects of the drug, whatever physical and emotional harm came from the abortion, and a dead child.

There are those, of course, who would argue that much valuable knowledge was gained. But at what price? And why? The price was 14 lives lost and 14 more damaged. The reason, in the end, is profit. What benefits the public medically, benefits the drug company financially.

Another type of fetal experiment was reported, in which it was difficult to find any reason that could even masquerade as noble.[64] The report came in a newspaper in Ireland in 1983, and was in reference to fetuses being used in the cosmetic industry in Europe. Experimenting on live fetuses had become part of the beauty product industry. Fetuses between the ages of 12 and 21 weeks were delivered alive by means of hysterotomy. Some of these children were then dissected and some of their internal organs were frozen. Other fetuses are frozen whole for later use. I find it hard to think of something so barbaric as being in any way noble. There is no excuse that can be offered for the murder of unborn children in the interests of smoothing the wrinkles and brightening the cheeks of the wealthy.

The preceding case — and, indeed, practically every case of fetal experiment — carries with it the threat or the actuality of a lucrative traffic in fetuses. This was also brought out in the report in Ireland in reference to Europe. The same abuse, however, is just as much a problem in the United States. In 1972 a witness at the Shapp Abortion Law Commission Hearing in Pennsylvania testified to the

---

[64] Cf. Rini, *op. cit.*, pp. 33-34.

reality of this trafficking.[65]   The witness had been an anesthetist for abortions at a hospital in Pittsburgh.   She spoke of how repulsive it had been to her to see aborted babies, still alive and trying to move and breathe, being packed in ice to be rushed off to some laboratory. The case mentioned earlier of the container full of fetuses (all belonging to just *one* pathologist) also bears witness to what a booming business this sort of activity may become. I suppose, however, it should come as no surprise that those who are willing to kill for profit will also be content to make still more money on the corpses of their victims.

There was one case of which Doctor Frankenstein himself might have been ashamed.  This took place in Finland in 1973, although the two doctors who conducted the experiments were from Cleveland.[66]  This time 12 fetuses were used, all of them between 12 and 20 weeks of gestational age.  They, too, were delivered by hysterotomy. (You may note that hysterotomy is favored because it produces a live fetus.) The heads were cut from the bodies and the internal carotid arteries were used to introduce a liquid medicine containing various substances. A carbon dioxide and oxygen mixture was used for balance and the material was retrieved from the veins and subjected to examination.

If you examine the sorts of experiments that have been done, you end up with a catalogue of horrors.[67]  Embryon-

---

[65] cf. Rini, *op.cit.*, p. 81.

[66]cf. Dr. and Mrs. J.C. Willke *Abortion:   Questions and Answers*, Hayes Publishing Co., 1985, P. 198.

[67] Detailed cases are given by both Rini and Willke.

ic tissue is used to attempt to grow organs. Brains, lungs and liver are removed from still living fetuses. One doctor cut open the rib cages of living children in order to examine the action of the heart — and some of these were as old as 24 weeks and, therefore, viable. Brains, hearts and other organs — sometimes taken from live fetuses — have been used for research or pesticides.

All I have offered here is no more than the tip of the iceberg. The list could go on and on. Why, you may be asking, have I chosen to offer you a catalogue of such gruesome and inhuman actions. I have done it as a reminder. Any of us can be caught up in causes that seem noble and humanitarian. We can easily be misled into thinking that the goal of helping humanity can be used to justify almost all that scientists want to do. This is especially the case when one's perceptions are further clouded over by sterilized and antiseptic language: hysterotomy, fetal tissue, products of conception. It all sounds so clean and scientific and official — until we face the fact that we are talking about tearing unborn children from their mothers' wombs and dissecting their still living organs. That is a cure for the one-eyed vision that so effectively distorts our view of reality.

We need to look not only at abstract goals, but at the concrete means used to attain them. We need depth in our vision. We must continue to realize that there is no such thing as a real "love of *humanity*" which can, at the same time, destroy *human beings*. It is a horrifying flat vision which learns to say, "I love humanity. Let me murder your children to prove it."

142

# CHAPTER 22

## WOMEN AND CHILDREN FIRST...

"Women and children first..." There was a time when that expression would have been the hallmark of chivalry. On that fateful night when the "unsinkable" Titanic struck an iceberg and began to founder, it was this statement which determined who should be first into the all too few lifeboats. This phrase would once have set the pattern for rescue operations from sinking ships, crashed planes and burning buildings. It has been the final utterance of more than one unsung hero. Alas! no longer.

"Women and children first..." is now quite likely to set the priority as to who shall first be exploited by science. Abortion has become fashionable. It is the "right" of every woman. And once so many women are willing to allow their unborn to be so easily and cheaply killed, something quite dreadful happens. Women become more depersonalized than they could ever have been in some of the former days of male chauvinism (a chauvinism which, by the way, I quite deplore). They now are viewed by many as the breeding grounds for experimental subjects and are persuaded to put their children to death under the pretext of serving humanity at large. Real people are sacrificed in favor of an abstraction.

It was the Supreme Court in its *Roe v. Wade* decision that gave national support to the dehumanization of the unborn and set the stage for the legal murder of 1.6 million of them each year. I can remember the first time I was called to an automobile accident and asked to minister to people covered with blood. It was not at all easy. Nor has it become easy. But you do learn to do it. Fortunately, since you are there to minister, you do not get used to or ignore the suffering, but you do learn to cope with it.

Some years ago I read (just when I cannot now remember) of an experiment that had been conducted to test the responses of people who were being asked to do something that they at first found distasteful. They were told they were part of an experiment in learning. They sat in a room at a desk on which there was a rheostat and a switch. They communicated with someone in another room and gave that person a test or a task to perform. The researchers told them that when a wrong response was made they should throw the switch, which would give the other person a mild shock. If mistakes were repeated, they were allowed to use the rheostat to give a slightly greater shock.

What happened was frightening. Most of those who controlled the rheostat were willing, after a while, to turn it high enough so that when they threw the switch they could hear the other person cry out in pain. Now the fact is that the person in the other room was not receiving a shock at all. The switch simply turned on a light and the supposed victim reacted accordingly. What was deplorable was the fact that people who at first were hesitant to cause pain soon became hardened to it. They were willing to inflict it in the interests of "science." In the interests of what they saw as some "higher good" they had become desensitized to the pain which they inflicted on others.

This desensitization is just what happens to those who become adept at torturing people as a means of interrogation. It is what happens to the many criminals about whom

144

we read each day — able to torture or kill for the sake of some negligible amount of money or property.

None of us should think that we are immune. The horrors of war, shown often enough on television, can become just another story to be watched while we eat dinner after a day at work. We can all become desensitized. Horrors first discovered make us ill. Horrors repeated more than a million times a year lose their power to arouse compassion and lead to a worse horror — the hardening of the human heart. Individuals become mere statistics and compassion fades into vague uneasiness and then into no feeling at all.

What then of 1.6 million abortions each year? That comes to 4,383 deaths *each day*. That means 183 per hour. *One every 20 seconds day in and day out, 24 hours each day.* The mind can hardly grasp what this implies. And so we can quickly lose interest. There are in the United States about 5,000,000 infertile couples, about half of whom will never have children of their own.[68] So many of them want to adopt, and still 3 children are purposely destroyed every minute of every day. And we become used to it. It is a "right." We are not allowed to interfere. In the end we may even find ourselves becoming bored by all the talk about it. We don't want to be "one-issue voters" — even though that one issue involves 1,600,000 persons cut in pieces and thrown away every year! There is hardly an issue more immediately threatening to human life.

The body of a 12 week fetus is only a few inches long. When laid out flat it takes up no more than 4 or 5 square inches. Even if all abortions were done at that stage of

---

[68] Cf. Barbara Eck Menning, *Infertility: A Guide for the Childless Couple*, Prentice Hall Press, 1977, 1988.

development (and many are done later) what would be the physical extent of 1,600,000 such tiny bodies? Packed side by side, in rank and file and pressed against each other, they would totally cover the full area of a football field so that not a blade of grass would be seen. And at twelve weeks these would be perfectly formed human bodies, needing only to grow in order to be able to live outside the womb.

How do the doctors and nurses who perform abortions overcome the horror of their own actions? How can they face the shredded arms and legs and crushed skulls? The fact is that many of them can't. They experience enormous emotional upset and begin to find the whole business so repulsive that they leave it.[69] It should also be pointed out quite clearly that my statements here are by no means aimed at all doctors nor at the medical profession in general. As of 1984 there were 300,000 physicians in the United States, only 8,700 of whom were willing to provide abortions.[70] That leaves 97% who are not willing.

The 8,700 seem to be able to conquer their human decency. They are surely desensitized and they are helped further with cold cash. The abortionist can work an easy week of 20 or 30 hours and earn up to ten times as much as a doctor who practices medicine. Indeed, back in 1974, when salaries were certainly not as high as they are now,

---

[69] Cf. Willke, *op. cit.*, pp. 191-193

[70] Cf. S. Hemshaw, "Competition Cutting into Case Loads," in *OB-GYN NEWS*, 1 September 1984: Cited by Willke, *op.cit.*, p. 193.

one Texas newspaper ran an add offering a *starting salary* of $180,000 yearly to join an abortion mill.[71]

The values of such people come to be centered in things, and persons will, perforce, become less and less important. There is no enthusiasm for new life. Such doctors take in and use people in order to improve their own positions. They are no longer real physicians caring for and saving human life. They are predators seeing to their own welfare.

How doth the little crocodile
Improve his shining tail,
And pour the waters of the Nile
On every golden scale!
How cheerfully he seems to grin,
How neatly spreads his claws,
And welcomes little fishes in
With gently smiling jaws![72]

The crass motive of money is not always admitted. There are, indeed, those who fancy themselves as rather humanitarian — while still making a good living. They will say they are involved in preventing suffering. Their motto may be, "Every child a wanted child." Not, of course, that *they* want them! They have no intention of helping people to accept children — there's no money for them in that. In plain English, what they really mean is, "Every unwanted child a dead child." And remember that these murdered children would have been born into a society in which infertility is ever more common and there is a waiting

---

[71] Cf. Willke, *op. cit.*, pp. 182-183.

[72] Lewis Carroll, *Alice in Wonderland*, 1865.

period of five years or more for those who want to adopt. Unwanted? Not at all. Simply unwanted by *this* mother at *this* time.

How about those who are willing to abort when the mother's life is at risk? They may be among the ones who have to act with reluctance. They are, however, still wrong. The direct killing of the innocent is not the way to save anyone's life. There are those also who will try to justify abortion in general on the ground of saving the lives of threatened mothers. Even if abortion were justified (and it is *not*) when the mother's life is at risk, that would account for less than 1% of all abortions annually. In *none* of those cases would it be *necessary* to abort the child and in many of them careful treatment would result in delivery safe to both mother and child.

Finally come the real "heroes" — those men of science who see 1.6 million dead children per year as an endless source of material for human experiment. As we have seen in preceding chapters, they are even willing, in many cases, to buy their deaths and conduct a flourishing business of trafficking in their bodies. They, too, like to think of themselves as humanitarians, spending themselves in the noble effort to conquer disease. Their times and talents are given over to experiments which lead to the advance of science. (Let us not dwell on the fact that they also lead to lucrative grants, fame and prestige. Such ignoble motives are, no doubt, purged from their altruistic minds.)

This last category brings up a question that we should look at more carefully. Is experiment on fetuses *ever* allowed? The answer is, "Yes, under certain conditions." These we will look at in the next chapter. For the moment let us consider only the question of experiment on *dead* fetuses. In general, there is no more objection to this than

148

there would be in the case of any autopsy. Back in 1976, when Father Thomas J. O'Donnell, S.J., wrote his excellent book *Medicine and Christian Morality*, he said:

> Some proposed regulations would prohibit teaching or research procedures on aborted fetuses, unless the abortion had been clearly spontaneous. While such a distinction would not be germane to the ethics of a Catholic hospital, it might concern an individual Catholic working in a public institution. Those who advocate the restriction seem to do so as an affirmation of the malice of induced abortion, or as a caution lest the desire for such fetal material prompt even more frequent abortion. Such reasoning seems inadequate. While restriction would limit valuable research, it is doubtful that the lack of it would encourage abortion. Nor is there any implied approval of crime in the use of autopsy materials derived from the bodies of those who have died as a result of murder or some other crime. Here again, of course, one must be aware of legal restrictions as well as the need for permission of the next of kin.[73]

In 1976 it seemed much less likely that research on dead fetuses would encourage abortion. However, the increasing need for fetal material in so many areas of research at present, and the willingness to pay, could most certainly increase the number of abortions. So, too, could the effort to justify abortion on the ground of the "good for humanity" in giving these "unwanted" persons over to use in science. At this point in our history, I would be less optimistic than was Father O'Donnell.

---

[73] Rev. Thomas J. O'Donnell, *Medicine and Christian Morality*, Alba House, 1976, p. 99.

In the *Instruction* this question of the use of dead fetuses is addressed. The document reads:

*The corpses of human embryos and fetuses, whether they have been deliberately aborted or not, must be respected just as the remains of other human beings.* In particular, they cannot be subjected to mutilation or to autopsies if their death has not been verified and without the consent of the parents or of the mother. Furthermore, the moral requirements must be safeguarded that there be no complicity in deliberate abortion and that the risk of scandal be avoided. Also, in the case of dead fetuses, as for the corpses of adult persons, all commercial trafficking must be considered illicit and should be prohibited.[74]

There is in the passage a clear rejection of the destruction of living fetuses. There is also a warning about the use even of those who are dead. The first warning is that there be no complicity in deliberate abortion. As we have already seen, such actions have indeed occurred. There is also the warning against the risk of scandal. It should be noted that the word "scandal" does not simply refer to the fact that some people might experience a sense of shock. It really means that we must avoid the risk of acting in such a way as to encourage people to do what is wrong. Those who speak of the need for research on fetuses are at times prone to justify abortion on the grounds that at least the murdered unborn are serving a useful purpose for humanity. That is surely scandal. In other words, research even on the dead can result in moral harm to the living.

---

[74] *Instruction*, n. 42.

In 1829 a man by the name of Burke was hanged in Edinburgh, Scotland, for murder. He was a "resurrectionist." This was the name given to those who made a living of robbing graves in order to sell the cadavers to medical colleges and hospitals. Burke added an extra touch. When fresh bodies were scarce, he simply made his own. In fact, if you consult a dictionary you will find that he gave rise to a new word in the English language. To "burke" someone means to kill by suffocation in such a way as to leave no trace. The market for bodies created a new industry.

We have to realize that the market for fetuses — dead or alive — does exist. It encourages abortion, because it adds another profit margin. Perhaps the day will come when we will have another new verb. To "pro-choice" someone may mean to murder him before he even has a chance to be born.

What of the living? What conditions or principles are involved? We shall look at these in the next chapter. In the meantime, don't be too anxious to step forward when someone says, "Women and children first..."

# CHAPTER 23
## "MAY WE HAVE A VOLUNTEER?"

The magician comes out onto the stage with a saw in his hand.  He waits as a coffin-like box is wheeled out on a platform.  With a flourish and a drum roll, his assistants whirl the box around so that you can see all sides of it.  There is silence and the magician says, "May we have a volunteer?"  The members of the audience all point to you and offer your services.  Of course, you might find that upsetting.  On the other hand, it is just an act, after all, so what do you have to lose?

What if it weren't an act?  What if the magician has no tricks up his sleeve, but is just testing a theory that he can cut you in half and — quite probably — put you back together again?  I don't imagine that you would be clamoring to get up on that stage.  Now suppose this were all for real.  Would you simply go along with it?  Would you feel that the audience had the right to volunteer you?    J u s t when are we justified in taking part in an experiment?  And when, if ever, are we justified in volunteering someone else to take part?  And — most germane to our present consideration — when are we justified in allowing the unborn to become subjects of experiments?

In the middle of the last century the hot item for politicians and for the whole country was the question of slavery.  As states were admitted to the Union, would they be slave or free?  One rallying cry for the pro-slavery group was "Popular Sovereignty."  Let the people choose!  It is, in

152

fact, just another form of the slogan, "Pro-choice." Each state, by election, should make the choice for itself. There you have it — the typical model of the traditional American sense of freedom, rights and fair play.

This was the position of Stephen Douglas in the debates with Abraham Lincoln. In one of those debates Douglas is reported to have said, "Every man should have the right to choose for himself if he wants to own a slave or not." Lincoln's response was, "You are in favor of a choice for everyone except for the person it matters most to — the slave."

The parallel between that situation and our own is so evident as to need no elaboration. In abortion the only one who is *never* consulted is the one who will be murdered. The same is true when it comes to experiment on a fetus. The unborn child is nobly volunteered by the mother who doesn't want him, the doctor who doesn't mind being paid to kill him, and the researcher who can hardly wait to get his hands on the body. All of this, of course, is in reference to situations in which the fetus is to be murdered in the act of abortion or later on in the experiment itself. Are there, however, other kinds of experimental procedures which could be morally acceptable? And, if so, what moral principles are involved?

The best way to examine this question is to begin by looking at what principles are involved when an adult is to be the subject of an experiment. This will help to clarify the way in which such principles can then be applied in the care of the unborn — or the case of anyone who cannot decide for himself.

The first point is in reference to the value and meaning of human life. It is at this point that the Christian and the "humanitarian" will differ. Those who claim to be humanitarians may mean that each human person is intrinsically valuable. Each one is worthwhile and is not to be exploited. Others, of course, may mean something quite different. For them it is "humanity" which has worth and value. The individual person (with the exception of themselves, of course) is expendable in service to "the race." The first group may or may not have regard for the unborn, depending on how they define human life. The second group may sound altruistic, but the fact is that they have no regard for anyone, child or adult.

The Christian begins with the realization that no human being has an absolute ownership over the life of anyone, not even over his own. Life is a gift of God and our control over it is one of stewardship, not full dominion. We are to cherish it, care for it and hand it back to God, its owner, when He asks for it. This implies, therefore, that we have not only rights but responsibilities as well.

We have no right to destroy our own lives and we have no right to take the life of any innocent person. We have, therefore, no right to enter into an experiment which will kill or which will cause serious bodily or mental harm. Nor do we have the right to experiment in any such way as to cause that sort of harm to anyone else.

Since we have this obligation for ourselves and our own lives, we then have the right to know what will happen in an experiment so that we are capable of making free and knowing choices in respect to our lives and welfare. This means that we have a right to be fully and properly informed about both the necessity and the possible consequences of any experiment in which we are asked to be engaged. Only in this way can we have the information that we need in order to make a good moral judgement. When the risks are appropriate and we see no danger of

154

serious harm or death, even then we must be free to decide whether we wish to participate or not.

It should be clear that no one has the right to volunteer someone else for experiment. That goes for adults and it most certainly goes for the unborn or for any of the other categories of persons who, for whatever reason, are unable to make free choices for themselves.

This full and informed consent is, therefore, essential in order to make moral decisions possible. There are also some facts about the experiment itself which can be put into the form of principles:

1. The knowledge sought through research must be important and obtainable by no other means, and the research must be carried on by qualified people.

2. Appropriate experimentation upon animals and cadavers must precede human experimentation.

3. The risk of suffering or injury must be proportionate to the good to be gained.[75]

There is another factor which should be taken into account when making decisions about participating in experiments. This is the difference between therapeutic and non-therapeutic procedures.

The therapeutic procedure is one in which the experiment is undertaken with the hope of improving the health of the person who acts as subject of the experiment. Such would be the case, for example, if someone with cancer decided to undergo an experimental treatment in the hope that it might help or restore his health. In this instance the treatment is not only an experiment, it is also a form of therapy.

---

[75] Benedict M. Ashley, O.P., and Kevin D. O'Rourke, O.P., *Health Care Ethics*, St. Louis, 1982, P.245.

The non-therapeutic experimental procedure is one which is done for the sake of knowledge, but has no beneficial effect on the person who serves as subject of the experiment. For example, a perfectly healthy person might be asked to take an experimental drug in order to see how it would affect his system.

When an experiment is therapeutic, a person may be justified in taking even serious risks. If it is a matter of an illness for which there is no tried and true remedy, and there is available an experimental and not yet proven remedy, one *may* make a morally good decision to undergo the experimental treatment. This is surely the case when the disease is life-threatening or even terminal, and the new procedure is risky, but really poses no threat greater than the threat of the disease itself. Obviously this also means that you would not be justified in undergoing an extremely risky experimental cure for a disease that did not pose much of a threat. The more serious the disease, the more serious may be the risk you can run to overcome it.

You are not justified in taking very serious risks for a non-therapeutic experiment. In this case you are really trying to weigh the good of an individual against the common good of society.[76] We must never lose sight of the fact that the individual has unique and intrinsic value and is never to be seen as a mere means to the good of society. Rather, the common good should exist for the benefit of each individual. How can you tell if the risk has become too serious? If you are submitting yourself to a real chance of death or serious and even lasting harm, then you are going too far. Father O'Donnell indicates that you

---

[76] Cf. O'Donnell, *op.cit.*, p. 96.

have gone past the limit of what is morally acceptable "once the danger has reached that degree of seriousness which makes the experimental act cease to be one of administration [stewardship] and begin to be one of absolute ownership."[77]

Now what does all this mean when we apply it to the case of the unborn? It is obvious that the unborn is one in that category of persons unable to make moral decisions. The unborn are incapable of giving informed consent. Does this mean, then, that no sort of experimental procedure can ever be carried out on the embryo or fetus? Part of the answer is to be found in something called proxy vicarious consent.[78]

Vicarious consent refers to instances in which one person acts on behalf of another who is unable to act for himself. This is the kind of consent which is involved, for example, when the members of a family give consent for treatment on behalf of someone who is unconscious. This sort of consent must always be given for the good of the person who is not capable of making the decision. Consent to experiment cannot be given in this way for the "good of humanity" or "the good of science" or even for the good of some other person. This would turn a person into an object to be used for others.

The first thing that is implied here is that we should not give consent to fetal experiment when it is non-therapeutic. In this regard, there are some moral theologians who would say that such consent could be given if the risks

---

[77] O'Donnell, *op.cit.*, p. 96

[78] Cf. Ashley and O'Rourke, *op.cit.*, pp. 248-250.

were truly minimal.[79]   Others would say that non-therapeutic experiments should not be done at all on the fetus.[80]
This would also be my opinion and it seems to be the
position taken in the *Instruction*, when it says:  "If the
embryos are living, whether viable or not, they must be
respected just like any other human person; experimentation
on embryos which is not directly therapeutic is illicit."[81]
Pope John Paul II has said:  "I condemn, in the most
explicit and formal way, experimental manipulations of the
human embryo, since the human being, from conception to
death, cannot be exploited for any purpose whatsoever."[82]

What about vicarious consent where we are dealing with
an experiment which is therapeutic?  No one has the right
to put the unborn child to death, nor does anyone have the
right to subject the unborn to the risk of injury or death for
the sake of science.  It is quite another matter if that unborn
child is suffering from something that brings it to danger of
death, and there is no safe or proven remedy.  What if we
do have a procedure still not fully tested yet offering some
real hope of success?  In that case parents can be morally
justified in allowing their unborn child to be part of what
is still essentially an experiment.

---

[79] E.g., cf. O'Donnell, *op.cit.*, pp. 98-99.

[80] E.g., cf. Ashley and O'Rourke, *op.cit.*, pp. 248-249.

[81] *Instruction*, n. 37. Note that the text uses the word "embryos" to refer to
fetuses as well.

[82] Pope John Paul II, *Address to a Meeting of the Pontifical Academy of
Science*, 23, October 1982:  *AAS* 75 (1983) 37 (cited in *Instruction*, ftnt. 29)

158

What makes this situation different? It is that here the procedure is therapeutic. It holds out some promise of real therapy, of healing. When a medical procedure is clearly therapeutic, then it may be allowed even for the unborn provided that no safer or proven way is reasonably possible. The purpose here is not the advancement of science or the acquisition of knowledge. Instead, the real purpose of the procedure is the honest effort to save the life of this actual unborn person. It is not something simply being done *to* the fetus; it is being done *for* him. It *does not create* a threat to life, but *attempts to overcome* a threat.

Pope John Paul II has said: "Any form of experimentation on the fetus that may damage its integrity or worsen its condition is unacceptable, except in the case of a final effort to save it from death."[83] The Congregation for the Doctrine of the faith in its *Declaration on Euthanasia* wrote: "In the absence of other sufficient remedies, it is permitted, with the patient's consent, to have recourse to the means provided by the most advanced medical techniques, even if these means are still at the experimental stage and are not without a certain risk."[84]

Parents can give consent to treatment necessary to save the life of their unborn child. No one, however, can or should give consent to the use of the unborn as animals for laboratory tests. We should never volunteer a human being

---

[83] Pope John Paul II, *Address to the Participants in the Convention of the Pro-Life Movement*, 3 December 1982: *Insegnamenti di Giovanni Paolo II*, V, 3 (1982) 1511 (cited in *Instruction*, ftnt. 31).

[84] SCDF, *Declaration on Euthanasia* 4 AAS 72 (1980) 550 (cited in *Instruction*, ftnt. 31).

— not even ourselves — as magician's assistants, even when the magic is called science.

# CHAPTER 24

## IMPOSSIBLE THINGS

*"There's no use trying," [Alice] said, "one can't believe impossible things."  "I daresay you haven't had much practice," said the Queen.  "When I was your age, I always did it for half an hour a day.  Why, sometimes I've believed as many as six impossible things before breakfast."*[85]

There are things which are impossible simply because they cannot be.  We have probably all heard the old question that school children would come up with in reference to the fact that God is all-powerful and infinite.  If God is able to do anything, then can He make a stone heavier than He can lift?  A real stumper.  If He *can* make the stone, then He can't lift it, so there is something He can't do.  And if He *can't* make the stone, then that is still something He can't do.  But don't we claim that *nothing* is impossible for God?

The answer, of course, is in a trick of language and in our own rather limited ways of seeing reality.  A stone (a finite object) which is beyond the power of God (an infinite Being) to move is a contradiction in terms.  Everything

---

[85] Lewis Carroll, *Through the Looking-Glass*, 1872.

161

created is finite — otherwise it would be infinite and, therefore, would be God. An infinite stone is a simple contradiction in terms — it is a juxtaposition of words without meaning when taken together. It is nothing — no thing. And, as we said, *nothing* is impossible even for God! Even God cannot make a thing which is not a thing.

You cannot have a circle with a circumference composed of four straight lines and four right-angled corners. The concept of "circle" eliminates "corners," and the concept of "straight sides" eliminates "circle." It is a case of joining of words in such a way as to eliminate any real possible meaning. In other words, some things are impossible because they simply cannot be.

There is, however, another category of things which can be, and yet we speak of them as impossible. What we mean is that there are actions so unthinkable that we are sure no one would ever perform them. They may be actions that seem insane or that are unspeakably cruel. No one would do such things. The fact is that we are all well aware that such "impossible" things happen every day. Just read the newspapers or watch the news on television. People are tortured; hostages are killed; atomic destruction is planned; children are abused, molested and destroyed. The unthinkable, the impossible, exists.

These things, however, are done by the demented, the unthinking, the uncaring. No honest, loving person could ever be guilty of them. Sad to say, this is not true. Even those who are, indeed, honest and loving and caring can be brought to do the unthinkable.

Do you recall the movie or the book called *Sophie's Choice*? A young mother, brought to a concentration camp by her Nazi persecutors, is forced to do the unthinkable. She is told that her two children will both be put to death

162

— unless she chooses one of them to be killed, and then the other will be allowed to live. A good and loving person forced to make an impossible choice. It was a choice that offered no alternatives that could be unregretted. It stayed with her for life, eating away at her until, in the end, she killed herself. It was the cruelest possible kind of choice, because it made love itself into a destructive force.

It was a situation built upon the unthinkable, the impossible. There was no right way out. It made for a powerful novel. Did such a thing ever happen? I don't know, but, if I were to judge by all I have read about the cruelty of the Nazis, then I must admit that it is a horror that could very well have occurred. How could anyone, even a Nazi, do such a thing? Quite simply, I regret to say. He would simply block out one essential fact, and then it all becomes quite possible. To him, Sophie was not human; she was a lower form of life, a non-person. What he did to her did not matter.

What is, in my estimation, most terrifying is that this sort of choice is now forced upon people regularly. It does not happen in concentration camps. It happens, instead, in fertility centers. It is not even done through mockery of love, but through a distortion of love — combined, of course, with the categorizing of some human beings as non-persons. It is not even done with the intent to be cruel, but it remains cruel nonetheless. It is possible because it is no longer unthinkable.

There are couples who long to have children and find themselves unable to do so. There are 5,000,000 such couples annually in the United States — about half of whom will eventually achieve pregnancy, while the rest will not. Those who are successful will often have gone through a series of examinations and treatments that may take months or even years.[86] They go to enormous trouble and expense in the interests of being able to bear a child of their own.

While the motivation for child bearing may have a wide range of possibilities, it would not surprise me to find that in the vast majority of cases the motive springs from the love that these couples have for each other. They long to share themselves and their lives with a child. They long to extend their love into the giving of life to a child whom they can love together. Their motives are good and worthy.

It would also not surprise me to learn that the vast majority of such couples are dismayed when they think of how many children are wilfully aborted. They are quite probably among the last people in the world who would think of hurting, let alone killing a child.

They spend time and energy and emotional strain and money — sometimes quite large sums of money — on treatments which tax budget and energy and human emotion, and even love, to heroic limits. Those couples who know right away that pregnancy is impossible (e.g. the man produces no sperm or the woman does not ovulate) have to cope with this hurtful news. Yet, in some ways, this may be easier than it is for those who have no idea why pregnancy does not occur. There are sperm, there are eggs. There is no evident problem with the reproductive organs. Still, pregnancy does not occur. Each month they try again. There seems to be no obstacle. Hope surges, only to be thwarted and end in disappointment which may become deeper and deeper.

---

[86] cf. Barbara Eck Menning, *op.cit.*, pp. xvii-xix, 3-8.

164

The simple examinations and possible cures come to an end, and the time arrives to try more complex techniques. These may begin with the milder sorts of fertility drugs, intended to cause multiple ovulation and thus to offer better chances of success. Stronger drugs are used, perhaps increasing also the possibility of multiple births if pregnancy should occur.[87] Finally, having exhausted all of the present ways in which it seems possible to aid in having intercourse result in pregnancy, the couple may be presented with further alternatives that begin to lead them inevitably to the need to make Sophie's choice.

The suggestion of *in vitro* fertilization may be next.[88] The method itself is simple enough in concept. The woman will be treated once more with a fertility drug designed to cause multiple ovulation. The results of this are not totally predictable, since they will depend not only on the effect of the drug but also on the woman's own hormone production and the condition of her ovaries. The hope is that there will be a number of healthy eggs produced, and that they can be successfully removed from the surface of the ovary by the physician. Actually, this can be done without any real problem, in most instances. The doctor will try to get between five and ten eggs — although in some cases as

---

[87] In a later chapter we will look in detail at the kinds of treatments now available and their moral implications. For now, I would simply point out that some methods -- but by no means all of them -- are morally wrong.

[88] The descriptions of the procedure involved in IVF are typical of what you will find in any book dealing with the subject. Some of the details in the text of this chapter, however, come from interviews with fertility experts as reported by Ann Wlazelek and Rosa Slater in the *Allentown Morning Call* of Allentown, PA (July 30, 1989, pp. Al, B20-B21; July 31, 1989, pp. D1,D2,D8; August 1, 1989, pp. D1, D6.

many as 25 have been recovered. With the man's sperm —
usually acquired by masturbation — they are fertilized in a
petri dish (a flat, plastic container, formerly made of glass
— in fact, the words "*in vitro*" are simply the Latin words
which mean "in glass"). Once fertilized, of course, they are
living human beings — each one a new person. They are
embryos in their first stage of cell division and development.

Usually only *some* of the new embryos are put into their
mother's uterus in the hope that all or some of those
selected will be able to implant. Already Sophie's choice
has been made, although the couple themselves did not
make it. *Some* of the embryos are given a chance for life.
What about the rest? There are various fates possible for
them. They may simply be destroyed. They may be held
for "donation" to another couple. They may be kept alive
for a time and used for experiment. They may be frozen
and set aside for later use — or eventual destruction. They
are human persons who are now doomed to be manipulated
as though they were mere objects.

What, however, about those which have been placed in
the uterus? Ordinarily about 8% to 10% may be expected
to implant —which means, of course, that it may take more
than one effort at IVF to lead to success. In most instances
only four to six fertilized eggs are put into the uterus at one
time — although in some cases more will be used. What
happens if all of them should implant (and this case does,
indeed, occur)? The more fetuses there are, the more
difficult will be the pregnancy and delivery. It is at this
point that the couple are faced with the nightmare of a
choice that cannot leave them without regrets.

I referred earlier to a process called "selective reduction."[89] It is also called "selective termination" or "selective abortion." The latter term is, of course, the most clearly truthful. In its most sanitized name it is known as "selective maintenance of pregnancy." In every form it means that someone is going to be killed.

One doctor explained the "ethics" of this in terms of the common good. He referred to it as a case of tragedy for the individual in order to produce betterment of the common good. In his view this meant that a baby would give up its life so that its brothers and sisters may live. This is a serious distortion of what is really meant by "common good."

The common good refers to a good held in common by all and serving for the benefit of all. "The common good is meaningless, except insofar as it protects and enhances the good of the individuals, who make up the community, whether that community be the Church, the State, or the World."[90] We cannot call upon the concept of the common good to justify the direct, purposeful killing of an innocent individual. It does *not* mean that we can randomly kill an individual in the interests of preferring the life of another individual.

There are cases in which people act heroically to save others, even though they themselves die in the process. "No one can show greater love than by giving up his life

---

[89] Cf. supra, chapters 6 and 7.

[90] O'Donnell, *op.cit.*, p. 16.

for friends."[91]  If someone freely tries to save the life of another and is shot and killed in the process, he may be a hero who acted out of love.  But his killer cannot then claim to share in the heroism and to have acted for the common good.  Nor can a terrorist lay claim to enforcing the common good when he kills only one or two of his hostages and turns over the rest unharmed.  In "selective reduction" the baby is not a willing hero.  He is a randomly selected victim of murder.  His killer is still a killer and not a medical hero of the common good.

The poor parents are forced into an impossible situation.  They must choose to save some of their children only by giving consent to the murder of others.  For the rest of their lives they must look at the children which survived and recall their part in the cost of that survival.  They are forced to live with a choice that was impossible.

There is an even further horror in all of this.  This procedure is often recommended when there are only three or four fetuses in the womb, on the ground (true in itself) that pregnancy and delivery are safer when there are only one or two.   This does not, however, mean that the delivery of three or four would have been a severe hazard.  And this is done even through any competent doctor could still care for and deliver all three or four, without serious risk to their mother.

There remains yet one thing which I want to say in reference to those embryos left in the dish and never put into the uterus.  It is a tragedy that these embryos, these persons, now referred to as "spare" embryos, are doomed to exist in a limbo of moral impossibility. *There is no morally*

---

[91] John 15,13.

168

*acceptable way in which they can be treated*! They are persons and should be treated with dignity and respect. Instead they are now offered the alternatives of being thrown away or frozen or used for experiment or being given away to other parents. They have no choice themselves and the only immediately available alternatives to those who control them are all wrong.

This is what is meant and implied when the *Instruction on Procreation* makes the simple statement: "In consequence of the fact that they have been produced *in vitro*, those embryos which are not transferred into the body of the mother and are called 'spare' are exposed to an absurd fate, with no possibility of their being offered safe means of survival which can be licitly pursued."[92]

---

[92] *Instruction on Procreation*, n. 45.

# CHAPTER 25

# WELL, I'LL BE A MONKEY'S UNCLE!

When I was growing up, one of the common expressions of amazement was, "Well, I'll be a monkey's uncle!" It's possible that it is an expression which dates back to the Nineteenth Century and the interest and satire which were both generated by Charles Darwin's theory of evolution. What is most amazing about our own Century is that that same expression may take on a whole new meaning. Instead of registering surprise, it may simply state a fact.

In the *Instruction on Procreation* we read the following: "Techniques of fertilization *in vitro* can open the way to other forms of biological and genetic manipulation of human embryos, such as attempts or plans for fertilization between human and animal gametes and the gestation of human embryos in the uterus of animals, or the hypothesis or project of constructing artificial uteruses for the human embryo. *These procedures are contrary to the human dignity proper to the embryo, and at the same time they are contrary to the right of every person to be conceived and to be born within marriage and from marriage. Also, attempts or hypotheses for obtaining a human being without any connection with sexuality through "twin fission, cloning or parthenogenesis are to be considered contrary to the moral law, since they are in opposition to the dignity both of human procreation and of the conjugal union."*[93]

It may seem to some that this is rather far-fetched and that there is no need even to worry about these sorts of problems. Who would ever think of attempting to cross-breed human beings with other species of animals? Why would there be an effort to put human embryos into the uteruses of animals? Why would we want to construct artificial uteruses? You may even be asking: "What is a gamete? What is twin fission or cloning or parthenogenesis?"

Let me begin by explaining some of the words that are being used. A *gamete* is a "germ cell." That is, it is a sperm or an ovum.

*Twin fission* refers to the process which seems to take place naturally when a single fertilized egg, at some point in its development, turns into two separate beings who will be born as identical twins. At present, of course, there seems to be no way in which we can cause this to happen. But it may well come about that it can be artificially stimulated.

*Cloning* refers to a process of taking a single cell from an already existing living being and causing it to develop into an identical individual. This could be done, for example, by taking the nucleus from a cell of an animal and transplanting it into an ovum whose own nucleus has been removed.[94]

---

[93] *Instruction on Procreation*, n. 46.

[94] Cf. Ashley and O'Rourke, *op.cit.*, p. 325.

*Parthenogenesis* means "virgin birth." In the case of an animal this would probably mean finding a way to stimulate the ovum so as to cause it to develop into an embryo without making use of sperm.

If you think about the questions I posed above, it will probably not take very long to come up with some reasons why people should try to do these very things. For example, in regard to the development of an artificial uterus, there might well be cases in which a fetus is unable to survive in its mother's womb and could possibly be kept alive until viability in some sort of artificial milieu. That could, I would think, be one case in which the use of such a device could be morally justified. There would be those, of course, who would see this as a way in which to avoid the discomforts of pregnancy — a use that would not be moral, since it would deprive the child of the relationship to his mother to which he has a right. There would also be those, we can be almost certain, who would see such an artificial uterus as an ideal way in which to breed or experiment on living fetuses. That, too, would be clearly immoral.

The transplanting of human embryos into the uteruses of animals could be envisioned for the very same reasons that one might want to construct an artificial uterus — and there would be the very same moral problems.

Cloning and parthenogenesis might be seen as ways in which to manipulate human nature itself by producing what the experimenters would envision as some sort of special or super race. The fact that it would be done without relation to sexual reproduction would also remove it from the areas of human love and warmth, from the essence of human procreativity. This, too, would be immoral.

172

In some ways, perhaps, the cross-breeding of species might seem to many to be the most outrageous of all the ideas mentioned. On the other hand, it might well be that this is the one area which currently presents the most likely chances of success as far as science is concerned. I am not aware of current experiments going on in this area at the level of human life, but there is certainly such work being done at lower levels.

Direct cross-breeding of different species is, of course, not really possible. The genetic structure of each species is so different from that of others as to make it impossible to fertilize the ovum with the sperm of another — at least, if neither the sperm nor the ovum are genetically altered.

There has, however, been enormous interest in the possibilities of recombinant DNA. Deoxyribonucleic acid (DNA) is a protein substance found in the nuclei of living cells and is the material in which are stored all of the specific and individual genetic characteristics of species and the individual member of that species. It is DNA which is responsible for the transfer of genetic characteristics from one generation to the next.

The restructuring of inherited characteristics by manipulation of the DNA has already been done in lower life forms and has, even at this stage, resulted in problems both real and potential.

Scientists have been able to change one-celled organisms in such a way as to give them new characteristics — in effect, producing a new life-form. But how can we even begin to predict what impact these life forms will have on others? Geneticists are now able to produce combinations of genes that may give rise to new species — and there is already discussion on the question of the legal complications involved in issuing patents on those new species!

Why, you may ask, would anyone want to patent a new life form? A little reflection will give you the answer. Suppose it were possible to invent a new kind of animal with commercial use? Or a new strain of plant that would revolutionize agriculture? The inventors — and investors — would expect a return on their work and their investments.

This may sound to you like science fiction, but, believe me, it is not. In July of 1989 the federal government gave approval to a New York state research institute to begin open-air testing of an altered virus.[95] The purpose of the new virus was to act as a pesticide which would do its job and leave behind none of the harmful residue that is so characteristic of chemical products. (Here is clearly a life form with the potential of profit.) The virus was to be tested on cabbage plants afflicted with the larvae of the cabbage looper.

The new virus (called *autographa californica nuclear polyhedrosis virus*) has considerable advantages. First of all, it attacks insects but does not attack vertebrates, so mammals (ourselves included) would be safe. Of course, this might well mean that other insects would not be safe. Once it had done its job on the intended pest, could it not move on to other insects? The intent of its inventors is to alter another gene in such a way as to prevent this. A virus protects itself with a sort of coating that surrounds it. The alteration of the gene would cause it to lose this protection. It would thus live for a few days, enough to do its work, and then be gone. (Of course, no one knows if it might be

---

[95] Cf. James C. McKinley, Jr., "Tests of Genetically Altered Pesticide Allowed," in *The New York Times*, Thursday, July 6, 1989, p. A13.

174

possible for it to recombine with other naturally occurring viruses and thus reacquire its protection.)

Surprisingly, the Environmental Protection Agency allowed the test, although, in fact, no one knows what may happen. If it does reacquire its normal protection, then it could go right on killing other insects. I must admit that when I feel something squishy crawling on the back of my neck, I am just as inclined as the next person to swat it. But any serious threats on insects in general would be a threat to us as well. What, for example, would be the effect on plant pollination if bees were attacked? And what of the myriad other things that insects are responsible for in the food chain and the balance of nature?

Of course, that is the story of a virus, not a human being. In May of 1989 it was reported that a step had been taken to clear the way for human gene transplant.[96] A decision by a judge in a Federal District court in Washington, D.C., determined that the National Institutes of Health must in the future hold in public the deliberations and votes of its Recombinant DNA Advisory Committee. This committee had given approval to the use of a foreign gene in an experiment to be conducted on ten patients with melanoma (a form of skin cancer). The article contains the interesting statement: "Only the health institutes can approve experiments to change the genetic makeup of humans."

---

[96] Associated Press release dated Washington, May 16, in *The New York Times*, Wednesday, May 17, 1989.

In March of 1990 there was still another report of gene therapy on human beings.[97] The Institutional Biosafety Committee of the National Institutes of Health held a public hearing and gave its approval to a plan to treat children with a severe genetic disease through the insertion of new genes into their blood cells. The disease with which they were concerned was Adenosine deaminase deficiency (ADA deficiency). This is the disease which attacks the immune system and was the subject of a great deal of publicity some years ago in reference to the boy in Texas who was forced to live in a plastic bubble to protect himself from infections or disease. This was seen as an indication that it would become possible for doctors to introduce into patients who lack it any sort of necessary gene.

The instances mentioned seem to be morally acceptable in so far as they are intended as therapeutic and are for the good of those who are undergoing such procedures. As to the degree of risk, I do not know enough about it so as to be able to make a judgement. What is thus far being done *may* be quite right. It would be naive of us, however, not to realize just what a Pandora's box is being opened.

Notice, that none of the cases I have referred to deals with the cross-breeding of humans with other species. What I am pointing out, however, is that gene manipulation becomes increasingly sophisticated and has left the realm of simple experiment on one-celled organisms. All of these cases, however, would not so long ago have been found only in the volumes of science fiction. Now they are here for real.

---

[97] Natalie Angier, "Gene Implant Therapy is Backed for Children with Rare Disease," in *The New York Times*, Thursday, March 8, 1990.

Not so many years ago I attended a lecture given by Arthur Clarke (the author of *2001*), in which he spoke of things to come in the area of science. He said that he had already heard of a plan in China to experiment on human and chimpanzee cells. The chimpanzee is, I think, our closest living relative as far as DNA is concerned. The intent of the experiment was to alter the genetic structure of either or both gametes in order to produce a new species of strong, docile and not overly-intelligent workers. (I suppose that you could also pay them in bananas and add to the potential profit.) The idea sounds insane, but do you really doubt that there are scientists who would be ready and willing to work on it?

The *Instruction on Procreation* is offering a warning. If we try to base our judgements on the morality of science only on the acquisition of knowledge, then we must be ready to proceed in any direction at all. Instead, we must never lose sight of the values of life and love and human interrelationship. We must not ignore the value of persons and focus instead only on our power to manipulate the world. If we do so, we could end up destroying what we claim to care so much about — human life. And we really could end up being monkeys' uncles.

177

In September of 1989 Judge W. Dale Young, in the Circuit Court for Blount County in Tennessee, made an eventful decision. After hearing the case of *Junior I. Davis v. Mary Sue Davis*, he decided in favor of Mary Sue Davis. The dispute was in reference to the fate of seven embryos — seven living human beings — frozen in liquid nitrogen at the Fertility Center of Eastern Tennessee.

The couple had undertaken the process of *in vitro* fertilization. Eggs had been removed from Mrs. Davis' ovaries and had been fertilized with Mr. Davis' sperm. The embryos had been allowed to grow and were then frozen and stored to await their placement in Mrs. Davis' uterus. In the meantime, however, Mr. and Mrs. Davis were divorced. They were now involved in a trial to determine who would have custody of the seven embryos. Mr. Davis wished to destroy them, on the ground that he and his wife were no longer married and that he could not be forced to become a father against his will. Mrs. Davis wished to have the embryos implanted in her womb so that she could have children. She and her lawyers contended that the embryos were human beings with rights. The other side contested this.

When the trial came to its conclusion, Judge Young ruled in favor of Mrs. Davis on the ground that: "From fertilization the cells of a human embryo are differentiated, unique

and specialized to the highest degree of distinction...
Human life begins at conception."[98]

One of the key witnesses in the trial was Doctor Jerome
Lejeune.[99]  In the remainder of this chapter, apart from
what is attributed to other sources, much will come from
Doctor Lejeune's testimony on August 10, 1989, before
Judge Young.[100]  In the course of his testimony he was
asked, "What ethical considerations do you  have about
freezing?"  In his answer, he said, "I think love is the
contrary of chilly.  Love is warmth..."

The process under discussion was cryopreservation, which
refers to the freezing of a living being in order to preserve
it — usually with the intention of bringing it back to its
original state of life.  It is a process being used now — as
it was in the case of these seven embryos — to keep
embryos alive but arrested at the early stages of development, when there have been only a few cell divisions. In
fact, the stage at which it is ordinarily done is when the
embryo reaches the size of eight cells.[101]

At this early stage of development the embryo is referred
to by some as a "pre-embryo."  This is still one more

---

[98] Reported by Ronald Smothers in *The New York Times*, September 22,
1989.

[99] Doctor Lejeune is a geneticist known throughout the world for his work
on hereditary chromosomal defects.

[100] The transcript was taken by the court reporters, Peggy M. Giles, C.C.R.,
Knoxville Court Reporting, P.O. Box 9112, Knoxville, Tennessee 37940.

[101] Cf. Barbara Eck Menning, *op.cit.*, p. 87.

example of the sanitized language to which I have referred earlier. It is used by those who favor abortion or are attempting to justify various kinds of manipulation of human life in its earliest stages. When Doctor Lejeune was questioned in regard to the "pre-embryo," he said that there is no such thing. There is either an embryo or not. He described it as a term invented by some British colleagues to give the impression that the first few stages of development involved something other than a human being. He described it as a change in words so that it would make it easier to justify a change in behavior toward the unborn. He said, "I think it's important because people would believe that a pre-embryo does not have the same significance that an embryo [has]. And, in fact, on the contrary, a first cell knows more and is more specialized, if I could say, than any cell which is later in our organism." In other words, in cryopreservation what is being frozen, even at the very first stage of cell division, is a human being — a human person.

You may be wondering just how it is possible to freeze a live being and then restore it to life. We think, sometimes, of such things as frozen food, meat for example, which surely could not be revived. The temperature of a frozen embryo is, in fact, even colder than that of frozen meat. When Doctor Lejeune explained what is involved in this process, he found a way to make it very clear and easy to understand.

The words "tempo and "temperature" are related in language. Both concepts can help in grasping the idea of freezing and reviving a living being. Atoms and molecules are in constant motion, and the tempo of that motion is related to temperature. Movement increases in heat and decreases in cold. The frozen embryo is a very tiny being, only about eight cells in size. Those cells are full of life

180

and they grow and develop at a tremendous rate, especially at the beginning. If they are gradually cooled, the motion of molecules and, therefore, their rate of growth will slow down. With the use of liquid nitrogen the temperature can drop enormously and then be kept down to minus 180° or 190° celsius. If this is done with sufficient care, the cells will slow down until time almost stands still for them and they are in a state that could be described as suspended animation. There is, however, a serious risk that the frozen cells may crystalize. If they do, then the embryo is killed. Gradual raising of the temperature should reverse the process, if the freezing has been successfully accomplished.

Even when the freezing is done in the most careful manner, there is still considerable risk. In the case of the Tennessee embryos, the embryologist who did the freezing (and who was named, quite appropriately, Doctor Shivers) testified that almost 30% of those frozen are accidentally killed. This is to say that about one out of three of these persons die, even in the care of experts. There are, of course, those who would say that even in the course of the natural process of reproduction there may be that many embryos which die. They would use this as a justification for taking this risk, even knowing that one-third will be lost. As I mentioned before, however, that is a very poor argument. We all know that 100% of all adults will die, but that would not justify us in subjecting a group of adults to some process on the grounds that only one-third of them would be dead by the time the process was completed. Indeed, it would be the process itself which had killed them. That would be considered totally unacceptable by legal and medical standards.

It is also worth asking ourselves this: When embryos are frozen, in whose interest is it being done? In the interest of the *individual* embryo? It would seem not. In the interest

181

of the couple who wish to have a child? It would seem so. Yet it is never right to risk another person's life in the interest of someone else, no matter how noble those interests may seem to be. I cannot turn another person into a means to my own ends.

The freezing of embryos at this early point of development is also justified by some on the grounds that the embryo at this stage is so incomplete that it could not possibly be considered human. I have responded to such objections in preceding chapters, but I found it quite interesting to read Doctor Lejeune's testimony in this regard.

What is present in the fertilized ovum or even in the first few cell divisions is *not* just human tissue or undifferentiated cells. In the laboratory cells (tissue) can be taken and made to grow, to reproduce themselves. But that is all that they do. They reproduce cells only of their own kind. Nerve cells will produce more nerve cells, skin cells will produce more skin cells. They will *not* produce a new individual, a child. The fertilized ovum, that new single cell which is called a zygote, if allowed to grow, will become a fully developed human being.

In other words, the fertilized ovum is an enormously complex being, containing in itself the whole genetic code of the individual. But it contains even more than that. It contains the whole pattern of development of all future cells and structures. It is, indeed, the *most* differentiated of all human cells. Even its mode of growth is unique. Tissue cells grow in multiples of two. One becomes two, two become four, four become eight, and so forth. The zygote, however, becomes two and then *three*. It will then become four cells and from then on it continues in multiples of two.

What is the significance of this peculiar deviation from the ordinary rules of cell division? The cells in these earliest stages are contained in a sort of covering called the zona pellucida. At the age of about six or seven days, when much cell division has taken place, the embryo "hatches" from the zona pellucida and develops so as to be able to implant. By that time the cells have indeed started to become different sorts of tissue, but the extraordinary dynamic of cells to become new individuals has been lost. Single cells can no longer be taken and cultured and grow into new persons.

In experiments with mice it has been found that cells from two mouse embryos can be taken from the zona pellucida and placed together in a third zona pelleicida whose original occupant has been removed. In some cases these have formed a new individual. Thus cells from the embryo of a white mouse have been mixed with cells from a black mouse and have, in some instances, developed into a mouse partly white and partly black. The same has been done with cells of three mice, and a few of them have developed into offspring with characteristics of all three cell lines. However, with four or five or more cell lines, the experiment will not work.

One inference has been that it is somehow at the stage of division of the embryo into three cells that the message is communicated that this is indeed an individual and not just a growing mass of cells. With the arrival of the fourth cell, further development is into the differentiated tissue types of all further growth. In fact, by the time of "hatching" from the zona pellucida, the cells lines can no longer be mixed. What does this mean? For one thing it would seem to mean that the fertilized ovum already contains the most powerful messages of its own individuality and growth. After its third cell division that individuality is so defined

183

that all future growth is into the integral parts of the one individual.

Doctor Lejeune also spoke of something else quite amazing and of which, I would say, most people are unaware. The sperm and egg each contain twenty-three chromosomes which join to form the forty-six that each person must have. Yet each contributes something different as well. One would think that if you could join the nuclei of two sperm or two ova, you would have the full complement of chromosomes and a new individual would emerge. This has been tried with mice, and has been found not to work. But something quite strange did happen. If two sperm are used, what results is not a new individual, but the growth, instead, of tissue which looks like parts of the membranes and placenta which support the growing embryo — but there is no embryo! If two eggs are used, what results is tissue — there may be pieces of teeth, or flesh or toenails — but still no embryo! In fact, there have been cases of human beings when, for some reason, the ova in the ovaries of a virgin woman have begun to divide and what resulted was not an embryo, but bits of flesh or teeth or nails. In other words, not only is an embryo an individual, but even the contributions of its father and mother are unique and involve something more than just twenty-three chromosomes from each.

Humanity is present at the very beginning of life, at the moment of conception. Father and mother have each made quite unique contributions, which have resulted in a new human being. No combination of egg and sperm from any other animal will result in a human being. And no combination of human sperm and human egg will result in some other species. To say that the zygote is not human is to speak nonsense. That single-celled being is, in a way, the *most* human being of all, the *most* fully human cell of all.

184

Doctor Lejeune said that when he visits a new city, there are two places that he loves to see. One is the local university and the other is the local zoo. He said, "At the university I have very often seen very grave professors asking themselves whether, after all, their children, when they were very young, were not animals, but I have never seen in a zoological garden a congress of chimpanzees asking themselves whether their children, when they are grown, will become Universitarians." Science makes it more obvious every day that human life begins at conception and that the embryo is a human being, while people still try to find some way to deny what is increasingly ever more evident. And it is all in the interest of doing what they want to do, regardless of the facts. Even the seemingly highest of motives must yield to the facts.

Doctor Lejeune described the freezing of embryos as "putting inside a very chilly space tiny human beings who are deprived of any liberty, of any movement, even... deprived of time." Time is frozen for them, making them survive, so to speak, in a "concentration can." This is not the way in which *any* human being should ever be treated. The stated intent may be to help people have children. The reality involves manipulation and possible death (in fact, *certain* death for up to one third) — things to which no parent would want to subject a child.

Finally, *no one* knows for how long an embryo can remain frozen and hope to survive. In fact, all of the evidence of tissue freezing or animal embryo freezing makes it clear that there is a limit. Beyond that limit is death or severe damage. Yet there are those who do not hesitate to freeze embryos, and then argue about the "ethics" of how long they can be preserved before they should be used for research or simply destroyed! They are

185

like people who assassinate the characters of others and then feel remorse over their poor grammar.

The *Instruction on Procreation* sums it up: "The freezing of embryos, even when carried out in order to preserve the life of an embryo — cryopreservation — constitutes an offense against the respect due to human beings by exposing them to grave risks of death or harm to their physical integrity and depriving them, at least temporarily, of maternal shelter and gestation, thus placing them in a situation in which further offenses and manipulation are possible."[102]  The warmth of human love demands more than this!

---

[102] *Instruction*, n. 47.

# CHAPTER 27

# DESIGNER GENES

There was a time when one would have thought of denim as the fabric of the poor. It was tough, durable, a little scratchy when new, and, if you wore it without washing it first, it turned your shorts blue. But then, in the late Sixties and early Seventies, when denim became a symbol of the civil rights movement, it was suddenly fashionable. Calvin Klein, Jordache and others appeared on the scene and whipped the blue jeans of the poor right out from under them. They added some fancy stitches (worth a few cents of thread), saved on cloth (by making them so tight that you'd have to grease your legs to get into them) and began to charge so much that the poor could no longer afford them. Then they made them tattered and torn and faded — and raised the price again. Designer jeans had arrived!

If these were the only jeans that were ever tampered with, I would have no real reason even to bring up the topic. The poor would have lost a bargain, the rich would have found a new way to waste their money and the world would have gone on its merry way. There is, however, another type of gene tampering that cannot be so lightly dismissed.

We have already seen, in earlier chapters, references to *genetic screening:* It is possible, by means of techniques such as amniocentesis, to diagnose certain types of genetic defects, such as Downs Syndrome. It is possible to diagnose carriers of Tay-Sacks or Sickle Cell Anemia or

Thalassemia, and it is possible to learn whether developing fetuses are affected with those diseases. At present, once a positive diagnosis is made, there is still no cure for the disease. The genetic defect itself cannot be altered. The fetus is subjected to the risks of amniocentesis with no hope of benefit to itself. Instead, the parents are offered the choice of abortion.

There is also another type of screening which is done after the child is born. For example, there is a metabolic deficiency known as phenylketonuria (PKU) which is transmitted genetically. Shortly after birth a blood test can reveal its presence. In this instance the disease, which would ordinarily result in mental retardation, can be treated by simple changes in diet.

It is obvious that the moral implications of genetic screening in this last case are much different than they are in the others. First of all, the method of diagnosis by blood test of the already born child does not involve the risk which accompanies amniocentesis. Furthermore, a positive result does not end in a death sentence, but in treatment which can really benefit the child. The treatment does not change the genetic facts, but it does change the undesirable results. Since PKU does occur, and since it can be so easily treated, many states have made the testing of the newborn compulsory. None of this seems morally wrong.

There is, however, one problem that has emerged. It has been found that not all of those who test positively for PKU end up showing signs of retardation — even when not treated. It has also been found that in some cases the special diet may have actually done some harm.[103] I am

---

[103] Cf. Ashley and O'Rourke, *op.cit.*, p. 318.

not saying this in order to indicate that such testing programs are necessarily wrong. I am, however, pointing out how even a relatively simple effort at correcting genetic defects can have unforeseen complications.

What if it were possible in cases such as Downs Syndrome not only to diagnose, but also to treat a child still in the womb? And what if it were possible not only to supply treatment, but even to bring about some sort of genetic or chromosomal change? Here we are concerned not only with genetic screening, but also with what is sometimes referred to as genetic engineering. One of the first questions we should ask is, "Why?" What is the reason and what are our motives? Is it for the benefit of the unborn child? Is it for our own benefit? Is it for the sake of acquiring new knowledge? If a treatment — even one which involves genetic or chromosomal changes — is being done for the real benefit of the one who receives the treatment, then we know that we are at least on the right track morally. If the benefit is more certain than is the risk, then we have further evidence that we are doing the right thing. If the treatment has been tried and tested and proven, then we can be even more secure in our moral judgement.

The fact is that no such treatment currently exists, nor is one likely to in the near future. It is not impossible that one will be found, but the present state of our knowledge does not hold out much hope of imminent success. In fact, in this area of genetic and chromosomal manipulation, we are far from full knowledge. Some work has been done on simple organisms, but the more complex the organism being considered, the less we know. And there is probably no organism of greater chromosomal complexity than is a human being. Even in the relatively simple matter of diagnosing and treating PKU we have learned that we are still quite prone to error. Yet this is nothing compared to the challenge of what happens when we try to make changes directly in the genetic structure itself.

You may wonder just why I am looking at the moral implications of a treatment that cannot presently be performed. I am doing so in order to point out that there is no total moral opposition to procedures which could cause genetic changes. There is no objection to real therapy for the unborn, even in this area. On the other hand, there would certainly be serious objections to these and any other procedures when they were done not as therapy but to benefit someone else in place of the unborn or as experiments for the sake of further knowledge. They become even more objectionable when they carry risks out of proportion to their therapeutic benefit.

What then of genetic manipulations which are not even intended as directly beneficial to the recipients, but are totally in the line of experiment? What, for example, should we say about efforts to control genetics in such a way as to change the nature of humanity itself in some fashion? This is a still wider application of genetic engineering. I referred earlier to the moral consideration that should be taken into account in the sort of genetic engineering that produces new viruses for commercial uses. The application of such principles to humanity itself should be of even deeper concern.

There are various levels at which some sort of "engineering" can affect the life and structure of the individual human being or even of humanity itself.[104] We are al-

---

[104] Although I am not quoting directly from them, I am here and in what follows in this chapter making use of Ashley and O'Rourke, *op.cit.*, pp. 305-306, 327.

ready familiar with reconstructive surgery or organ transplants - either organs from another individual or bionics. The latter could be used not only to replace, but even to enhance present human capacities. In the area of embryology it is possible to intervene in such a way to cause changes in growth or development, even without altering genetic structure itself. We have seen cases of this, for the most part, in a negative sense. A mother who drinks alcohol or uses drugs in a pregnancy can, at various stages, make quite drastic changes in her child without any real genetic alteration. These changes can be extensive both physically and psychologically, as, for example, the changes which take place through fetal alcohol syndrome. It should be possible, if we knew how, to introduce in some cases of defective embryos drugs which could result in beneficial rather than harmful changes. Genetic engineering, however, opens up possibilities much more far reaching than these. In fact, genetic engineering holds out the theoretical possibility of such control over the genes as to make it possible to combine genes so as to produce individuals who are "made to order."

One type of genetic engineering which is already in process is the effort to predetermine the sex of a child. The chromosomes which determine gender are called X and Y. The letters don't stand for anything, but are merely based on the fact that the one chromosomes looks like the letter X and the other looks like the letter Y. The cells of females contain two X chromosomes and the male cells contain one X and one Y. When sperm are formed in the testes, part of the process involves cell division in which the usual 46 chromosomes of the human cell are divided so that each sperm (just like each egg) contains only 23. The X and Y are separated so that half of the sperm have an X and half have a Y. All eggs, however, contain only an X.

If a sperm with an X chromosome fertilizes an egg, the embryo will have two X chromosomes and will develop into a girl. If the sperm has a Y chromosome, the embryo will have one X and one Y and will be a boy.

It has been found that the sperm with an X chromosome seem to have a different density than do those with a Y. They can, therefore, be spun in a centrifuge and separated. Some have claimed a good percentage of success in determining the sex of a child by selectively using the sperm for *in vitro* fertilization. This has led also to the idea of finding methods to suppress the production of either X or Y chromosomes in the male, thus insuring the conception of a child of one sex or the other.

Is there anything wrong with this? At first glance, many might feel uncomfortable with it, but could also be hard put to explain just what it is that seems wrong. First of all, we might note that biologists see the natural process of sexual selection as a way in which nature assures that the distribution of the sexes will stay at just about 50-50. In fact, the conception rate of males is just a little bit higher than 50%, which, rather amazingly, offsets the fact that male embryos experience a slightly higher mortality rate.[105] Tampering with this natural process could have very undesirable effects in the long run. That, however, is not all that is at fault here.

Why would parents choose a child of one sex rather than the other? There is hardly any answer available except for a personal preference, possibly based on cultural biases. There is, however, an underlying factor in this whole question which should not be overlooked or treated lightly.

---

[105] cf. Ashley and O'Rourke, *op.cit.*, p. 324.

The manipulation and inevitable destruction of living embryos through *in vitro* fertilization, and the reduction of children to the status of objects of commercial transaction through surrogate motherhood, are both indications of an attitude which somehow begins to see children as the property of parents. This attitude is painfully evident in the abortion mentality which has become so pervasive in our culture. Children are more and more treated as objects of their parents hopes and expectations and less as persons to be accepted, loved and treasured in themselves. Ashley and O'Rourke say:

> Christian teaching shows that is a major significance to children that they be accepted by their parents as a divine gift to be loved for what they uniquely are and not merely because they conform to the parents' hopes or expectations. At the present time, society is becoming more aware of the immense injustice and harm done to women by culture patterns and structures which constantly say to a girl, "You should have been a boy." Sex selection by the parents will either reinforce this male preference pattern, or if parents can be reeducated to equal preference, it will still say to the individual child, "You are loved because you conform to your parents' preferences." This seems an injustice to the child and further reinforces the cultural message that children exist primarily to fulfill the needs of the parents rather than for their own sake. This implication is already built into many cultural structures, and people have an ethical responsibility to fight against it. The

health care profession should discourage such attitudes, not promote techniques to further them.[106]

There still remains a far more frightening aspect of genetic engineering. This is the possibility of using our knowledge of genetics to attempt to create "superior" human beings or babies "made to order." This might be accomplished by cloning. This would involve taking the nuclei from cells of an individual and planting them into an ovum whose own nucleus had been removed. This ovum would then be transplanted into a surrogate mother's uterus to grow into an identical twin of the original. Another method would be to recombine the genes in a zygote (a fertilized egg). This could be done by a process referred to as "transduction." This involves putting a portion of a chromosome into a virus which is then able to enter a human zygote and implant this new chromosome portion there. It may even become possible, in this way, to introduce chemically synthetic genes which do not now even exist. All of these processes open up avenues which lead further and further away from the value of the individual, and which open the more terrifying possibility of changing humanity itself. And every step in this direction would be at the cost of a trail of discarded, "spare," dead embryos as — the "failures" who fall along the way in the brave march of scientific "progress."

This sort of genetic engineering has implications not only for the individuals who are produced by it, but for the whole race. The new genes would become part of the "gene pool" incorporated into succeeding generations. It would be almost impossible for anyone even to begin to

---

[106] Ashley and O'Rourke, *op. cit.*, pp. 324-325.

194

predict what these new combinations of genes would bring about. The justification for taking such risks would probably be the eventual "improvement" of the human race. But who has the kind of knowledge that can determine just what improvements should be made? Alasdair McIntyre offers some suggestions as to what sort of people scientists might want to produce. His criteria are summarized by Ashley and O'Rourke:

They would have the ability to live with uncertainty; to keep rooted in the particularity of everyday life; to form nonmanipulative relations with others; to find their fulfillment in their work; to accept death; to keep hopeful; and to be willing to die for their freedom. He then concludes, "The project of designing our descendants would, if successful, result in descendants that would reject that project."[107]

The desirable aspects of genetic engineering are quite limited and are related to directly therapeutic goals. Even there they are, to a large extent, more than a little unpredictable. Non-therapeutic uses seem to carry with them enormous risks and no truly desirable ends. It is little wonder that the *Instruction on Procreation* says:

Certain attempts to influence chromosomic or genetic inheritance are not therapeutic but are aimed at producing human beings selected according to sex or other predetermined qualities. These manipulations are contrary to the personal dignity of the human being and his or her integrity and identity. Therefore in no way

---

[107] Ashley and O'Rourke, *op.cit.*, p. 307, referring to Alisdair McIntyre, "Seven Traits for Designing our Descendants," in *Hastings Center Report* 9 (1979): 5-17.

can they be justified on the grounds of possible beneficial consequences for future humanity.[108]

---

[108] *Instruction*, n. 48.

## CHAPTER 28
## LET ME HELP YOU WITH THAT...

It's Christmas morning and Santa, with his round little belly full of air-dried cookies and room temperature milk, has found his way back to the North Pole. The reindeer are unhitched, the sleigh is put away and it's time for Jolly Old Saint Nick to take off his boots, put up his feet and let visions of sugarplums dance through *his* head for a while. Does he realize that behind him he has left a trail of consternation, frustration and puzzlement such as no one was ever meant to face so early on the morn of a cheerful holiday?

Everywhere are opened boxes of not yet assembled toys — many of them doomed to failure even after assembly, since, of course, the small print says, "Batteries not included." In some homes patient parents explain to their children that part A should be attached to part B, using bolt 10 and nut 11. The work goes slowly, but both parent and child learn something — not only about mechanics but about each other as well, and a rather tedious process ends in a general sense of satisfaction.

Then there are those homes in which a father, after viewing the clumsy efforts of the child, says, "Let me help you with that..." The child, annoyed and bored, does nothing but hand over pieces called for by the father who — perhaps even quite skillfully — produces a toy just like the picture on the box. It is not the production of the child and he was not really helped. He was merely replaced.

There is a vast difference between assisting and replacing, although there may be points in the process when it is hard to tell which is actually taking place. In the case of assisting, the relationship of the makers is as important as is the relationship of the parts. Not so when one of the builders is replaced by the other, who needs only the plans and the parts and can make do quite well without any further help. Mutual endeavor is set aside in favor of getting the job done.

The origin of new human life should be more than just the coming together of ovum and sperm. The beginning of a life involves not just a relationship of cells, but a relationship of persons as well. Human beings should not just "breed." They should *procreate*. Babies should be conceived and born into a permanent and faithful marriage, because it is only within that sort of bond that they can be given a fair chance at developing into the fullness of life to which they have a right. In fact, when they are not born into that sort of union, society has traditionally tried to do something to rectify the situation. Adoption, for example, is one means of trying to supply the loving, familial environment that is lacking for some children, but that is present in a happy marriage. (This has, unfortunately, been overlooked in our own day and age, when we see adoption promoted for single parents or even for homosexual pairs.)

To be conceived and born into a union of love implies more than simply growing up as the child of parents who happen to love each other. Union is demanded in the conception itself. Sexual intercourse is not just a mechanical means of transferring sperm into a woman's body. It is an act of self-giving in which the bond of love, which is

198

both spiritual and emotional, is also expressed physically. Those emotional, physical and spiritual aspects form one whole, one living expression of love. Whenever we attempt to separate them, we do violence to the meaning of sex and we do violence to ourselves. Sexual promiscuity, for example, focuses on the physical and emotional pleasures of sex, with no regard for the spiritual aspects of personal union. As a result, it becomes destructive since it reduces persons to the level of objects. The person who is promiscuous becomes increasingly incapable of the sort of commitment and fidelity that make marriage possible — and it is only in marriage that sexuality assumes its real meaning.

The meaning of sex is also distorted when the emotion and pleasure which accompany it are misdirected. This is most obvious in those persons who find pleasure in pain and become caught up in sadism and masochism. Sex ceases to be procreative or unitive and becomes, instead, consciously and physically destructive. It has a destructive force also when its purposes are distorted in other directions. It may be used as a weapon by being withheld in a marriage, or it may be used as another sort of weapon in order to hold on to someone. It may be used as a physical or emotional shortcut to solving problems in a relationship — becoming eventually destructive simply because it never really does solve those problems. Indeed, it *cannot* solve them.

The whole area of artificial means of procreation is filled with the possibilities of turning sex into something damaging or destructive. This is why the Church is so concerned about it. In many instances the destructive force is subtle and its effects may not be at all evident at first. That, of course, is true in many of the destructive patterns that can be introduced into the context of sexual activity.

What, then, should we say to those who suffer all the pain of infertility? Is there nothing that they can do? Of course there is, and in the later chapters I will go into those possibilities in some detail. For right now, however, I am interested in pointing out some of the basic facts, from which basic principles are evolved. This makes it possible for us to be able to tell what means should or should not be used in the efforts of a couple to have children.

The *Instruction on Procreation* is somewhat limited in its point of view. This is a conscious and freely chosen limitation. The document is not intended to be a complete study of methods of overcoming infertility. It directs its attention, instead, to broader areas in which there are, indeed, moral problems.[109] Only near the end of its treatment of the topic does it set out the positive factors which point to some ways in which medicine can find moral solutions to this painful problem, but even there it does not describe specific answers.[110] So, for right now, I would like to begin with the general norms presented in the *Instruction*.

When the *Instruction* begins its examination of ways in which science and medicine intervene in human procreation, it points to the sort of destructive patterns that exist at present. It gets that out of the way first. It also limits its consideration to what it calls "artificial procreation" or "artificial fertilization." These terms are used to refer to methods or technologies that try to bring about conception in some way that is apart from sexual intercourse between

---

[109] Cf. *Instruction*, nn. 49-87.

[110] Cf. *Instruction*, nn. 85-96.

200

husband and wife.  In other words, the *Instruction* is going to deal with two topics primarily:  *In vitro* fertilization and artificial insemination.   There are moral problems with both.

The most obvious problem with *in vitro* fertilization is, of course, that the method itself *always* ends up causing more death than life.  I have spoken of this more than once in earlier chapters, so I will do no more here than to simply quote the document itself:

A preliminary point for the moral evaluation of such technical procedures is constituted by the consideration of the circumstances and consequences which those procedures involve in relation to the respect due the human embryo.  Development of the practice of *in vitro* fertilization has required innumerable fertilizations and destructions of human embryos.   Even today, the usual practice presupposes a hyper-ovulation on the part of the woman:  a number of ova are withdrawn, fertilized and then cultivated *in vitro* for some days.  Usually not all are transferred into the genital tract of the woman; some embryos, generally called "spare," are destroyed or frozen.  On occasion, some of the implanted embryos are sacrificed for various eugenic, economic or psychological reasons.  Such deliberate destruction of human beings or their utilization for different purposes to the detriment of their integrity and life is contrary to the doctrine on procured abortion already recalled.

The connection between *in vitro* fertilization and the voluntary destruction of human embryos occurs too often.  This is significant:  through these procedures, with apparently contrary purposes, life and death are subjected to the decision of man, who thus sets himself up as the giver of life and death by decree.   This dynamic of violence and domination may remain unnoticed by those very individuals who, in wishing to utilize this procedure, become subject to it themselves. The facts recorded and the cold logic which links them must be taken into consideration for a moral judgement of IVF and ET (*in vitro* fertilization and embryo transfer); the abortion mentality which has made this procedure possible thus leads, whether one wants it or not, to man's domination over the life and death of his fellow beings and can lead to a system of radical eugenics.[111]

However, what if it were possible to use *in vitro* fertilization without the destruction of the embryos? What if the risks were also drastically reduced? Would it then be morally acceptable? In other words, is the Church's moral objection to *in vitro* fertilization based only on the fact that lives are destroyed, or are there further problems?

There are, of course, further problems, but many find them harder to see, even though they may readily see the moral evil of *in vitro* fertilization as it is currently practiced. The additional moral problems will only be understood if we see the reality of procreation from a truly Christian point of view.

Marriage is the place in which children should be conceived and raised. Husband and wife choose to make a lifelong commitment to each other in love, thus creating a situation of loving union and stability which allows for true procreation of each other and of a family. This commitment is not simply "spiritual," without regard for the seemingly mundane material aspects of life. It must

---

[111] *Instruction*, nn. 50-51.

involve the spirit — the heart and soul of each partner — but it takes a material form as well. It involves earning a living for mutual support. It involves a place to live, caring for property, cleaning, cooking meals, taking care of each other in illness. It is the fullest sort of self-giving. Spiritual love becomes "incarnate" in such ordinary realities; and the rather commonplace aspects of worldly life are given depth of meaning by the spiritual dimension of love. When they are separated, love begins to die. We are creatures of body and soul, and both must work as one in the living of human life.

Procreation, in the Christian view, is a collaboration with God. Sexual intercourse, if it is what God means it to be, is a bodily expression of the fullest kind of human love and union. When it becomes less than that, it ceases to be what it ought to be. When it is reduced to the mere mechanics of breeding, then it has begun to lose its true meaning. This is what begins to happen when the creation of a child is separated from intercourse itself and becomes, instead, a technical process of combining egg and sperm in a laboratory. The parents may indeed truly love each other. They may long for a child of their own. They may have the best of intentions. Yet, once they begin to separate the begetting of a child from the physical expression of their love for each other, they begin a process that is contrary to real procreative love. Their child starts to become a product rather than a procreation. Their loving act is replaced by masturbation, egg retrieval and the work of technicians. Something begins to happen to their commitment to the self-giving in which they offer each other the right and the gift of becoming father and mother only in and through each other.

Sex in marriage should be both unitive and procreative.[112] The two elements are inseparable and neither of them should be destroyed or set aside. The sexual relationship of husband and wife is a concrete expression of their love and self-giving. Children should be conceived and born from that sort of loving act. Our bodies are not just objects that we can manipulate in whatever way we choose. Our bodies are ourselves. It is in and through the body that our loves and relationships come to life. The child, the most concrete expression of procreative and unitive love, should come into existence in and through that unitive act, and should never be viewed or treated simply as the product or outcome of purely physical components.

The child should be the result of an act in which father and mother express their loving union with each other, and not the product of the works of a technician. Parents may be tempted to say that their desire for a child comes from love and that they subject themselves to this technical process out of love. And indeed they may think so and want to believe so. But it is not a very good argument and we have all seen things done "out of love" that were not very good things at all. Depth of feelings, depth of desire and depth of loving may be very real, but they are all too often used as a basis for poor moral judgement. In this case they can lead a married couple away from the loving act of procreation through sexual union and force them instead to find themselves merely supplying the raw materials from which someone else will try to "make a child." What may seem a very good intention can find

---

[112] A far more detailed expression of what I am presenting here can be found in many of the chapters in *Reproductive Technologies, Marriage and the Church*. The Pope John Research Center, 1988.

itself becoming, instead, a potential source of failure in a relationship.

Then what can medicine and science do to help with the truly painful problem of infertility? Do they have any contribution to make that would be morally acceptable? Indeed they do; but that contribution is, perhaps, best understood by starting with a very simple outline of what is involved in the act of procreation.

The natural process of procreation seems to be easily understood in terms of three stages. The first is the act of sexual intercourse. The second is the process by which egg and sperm make contact in the body of the woman. The third is the fertilization of the egg by the sperm in the mother's body at the moment of conception. Procedures which ignore or set aside any of these three elements create moral problems.

Even if *in vitro* fertilization were not so totally linked with the death of embryos, it would still violate every aspect of those three elements. It totally ignores the conjugal act and its central place as the living expression of procreative love. It begins with no sexual act. An egg is removed from the ovary, sperm is taken by masturbation, and no real act of sexual love occurs at all. There is no bodily process of union of sperm and egg. They are simply put together in a dish where they fertilize and begin to grow. Every aspect of human conception is bypassed.

Problems with fertility may, indeed, occur at any of the three stages. Medicine may also attempt to correct problems at each of those stages. In each instance it has the potential to help and not simply to replace the natural act and process. In fact, it is here that we can find one of the most basic moral norms relating to treatment for infertility. It is this: Procedures which are morally acceptable will *not* replace the act or the process, but they will assist it or make it possible. Procedures which *replace* the act or the process are not morally acceptable. As we shall see in later chapters, there are procedures which do indeed assist without replacing. There are also some procedures about which moralists are not sure. Some see them as assistance and some see them as replacement. More about that later.

Fertility problems may occur at the time of intercourse itself. There may be a problem with ejaculation. There may be a problem of impotence. There may be a problem with the pH balance in the vagina. These and other problems can often be treated *so as to make intercourse possible*. There may be problems related to the meeting of sperm and egg. Tubal blockage may make it impossible. Sperm may not be sufficiently motile. Chemical imbalance may create a hostile environment. Ovulation may not be occurring. Here again there can be modes of treatment which make it possible to *assist the natural process or correct some deficiency*. Even when sperm and egg meet, there may be factors, such as chemical or enzyme problems, which interfere with fertilization. Once more there may be treatment which *assists in making natural fertilization possible*.

Frequently there are other factors to be taken into account, but in general we can safely say that a procedure which *assists* the natural act and process is going to be morally acceptable. A procedure which *replaces* the natural act or process will surely be morally unacceptable. The fact that something is technically possible does not mean that it will be therefore morally acceptable. It might be worth pointing out that the procedures which attempt to assist do not always work, but they also do no moral harm and are frequently unlikely to cause further physical harm.

206

*In vitro* fertilization does not always work (in fact, 90% of the time it *does not*), but it *always* causes moral harm.

All of the things of which I have written in this chapter can help one to better understand what the Church believes and teaches. The *Instruction on Procreation* points to it in a few brief sentences. In relation to conception, birth and parenthood it says:

> The child has the right to be conceived, carried in the womb, brought into the world and brought up within marriage: it is through the secure and recognized relationship to his own parents that the child can discover his own identity and achieve his own proper human development.

> The parents find in their child a confirmation and completion of their reciprocal self-giving: This child is the living image of their love, the permanent sign of their conjugal union, the living and indissoluble concrete expression of their paternity and maternity.[113]

In regard to the essential differences between assisting in or replacing the natural act and process, the *Instruction* says:

> It sometimes happens that a medical procedure technologically replaces the conjugal act in order to obtain a procreation which is neither its result nor its fruit. In this case the medical act is not, as it should be, at the service of conjugal union but rather appropriates

---

[113] *Instruction*, nn. 57-58.

to itself the dignity and the inalienable rights of the spouses and of the child to be born.[114]

Keep clearly in mind the distinction between assisting and replacing. It is important. Someone who really can assist you may be a blessing to you. Someone who begins by saying he can help you, and then replaces you, is not really thinking about you. He is simply "getting the job done." He may be helping you to breed. He is not helping you to procreate.

---

[114] *Instruction*, n. 90.

## CHAPTER 29

## A LITTLE LEARNING

In 1711 Alexander Pope published that masterpiece, *An Essay on Criticism*, in which are those lines familiar to every student of English literature and often quoted, at least in part, by those who do not even know their author:

A little learning is a dangerous thing;

Drink deep, or taste not the Pierian spring:

There shallow draughts intoxicate the brain,

And drinking largely sobers us again.

The sentiment expressed by Pope did not originate with him, in spite of the originality of his way of saying it. In the century before the birth of Jesus a Roman writer, Pubilius Syrus, had written as one of his *Maxims*: "Better be ignorant of a matter than half know it."

The lesson is clear and most of us have learned it by experience somewhere along the line — perhaps even more than once. You act on partial knowledge and are lucky if the only bad effect is embarrassment. It is a lesson that we all need, and it is a lesson that science and medicine seem to need to learn over and over again. We look back at the past and are shocked at the sorts of treatment that were dispensed by doctors. The medical practitioners of the Nineteenth Century looked at their predecessors and were convinced that their own time was the pinnacle of medical achievement. We look back to the last century, however, and marvel at how much they did *not* know. Then we promptly act on what *we* know, forgetting that the next century will probably be astounded at the way in which we survived our own primitive medical practices!

I do not mean to imply that we should do nothing, but I want to point out that we have to admit and accept our limits. The more important our area of concern, the more we should be aware of the need for caution. Nowhere is this more true than in problems related to infertility. We are dealing with human life itself and it deserves to be treated as serious and sacred.

The causes of infertility are sometimes evident, sometimes discoverable by examination and sometimes are never discovered. The fact is that in about 10% of cases of infertility our present methods of diagnosis reveal no apparent cause at all.[115] Even when the cause is discovered, this does not guarantee that the infertility can be corrected. Of the 5,000,000 infertile couples at present in this country, only about 50% will find that their infertility can be corrected.[116] Treatments which work for one couple simply do not work for others — and no one can really say why.

I mentioned earlier that some of the procedures used to "help" infertile couples are morally wrong. For this reason the Church, in its teaching, opposes them. Some of the procedures and the aspects which are immoral have been

---

[115] Cf. David S. McLaughlin, M.D., "A Scientific Introduction to Reproductive Technologies," in *Reproductive Technologies, Marriage and the Church*, the Pope John Research Center, 1988, pp. 52-67.

[116] Cf. Menning, *op.cit.*, P.xviii.

210

described in previous chapters. There are, however, some things which can be done to help the childless couple and which are morally acceptable. These are procedures which, in one way or another, truly do assist in the natural process of conception. In order to understand what these procedures are and how they work, it helps to know some of the possible causes of infertility and how they are diagnosed and treated.

In the normal course of events, a woman, from puberty to menopause, will have a menstrual period each month. That period signals the end of one cycle and the beginning of the next. Ideally, the period occurs every 28 days. Hardly anyone, however, coincides totally with the ideal, and menstruation is no exception. A woman's cycle may vary. Normal ranges may be as few as 23 days or as many as 34. In each instance, however, there is one factor that is rather constant. It is this: When the menstrual period begins, you can know that ovulation had occurred 14 days earlier. That, of course, regular as it may be, is of no help in telling you just when ovulation will occur next month. You could study a woman's cycle over a period of some months and you might be able to come up with a good estimate of just when the next ovulation will occur. But it would still be just an estimate.

Of course, there are some visible and easily detectable signs that can tell you — quite accurately — just when ovulation is taking place. There is a slight rise in basal temperature; there is a visible change in cervical mucus; some women can actually feel the egg being released. The method of observing and making an estimate was the basis for the old calendar method of family planning by means of rhythm. The use of temperature and mucus is the foundation for the present, very accurate, method of natural family planning — sometimes called the Sympto-thermal Method.

Both of these are also methods by which one can increase the chances of having a baby when there is some first indication of possible infertility.

When an egg is released from the ovary, it is drawn into the open end of the fallopian tube and moves slowly toward the uterus. For a period of 12 to 24 hours it is fertile. If it is entered by a fertile sperm, conception will take place. This should happen in the upper end of the tube, so that its slow journey to the uterus will allow it time for sufficient growth to make implantation possible. If egg and sperm are in the right place at the right time, conception will occur in about 1 out of 5 cases. In fact, if a couple are having intercourse during this fertile period of the cycle, and if they are not using contraceptives, and if they continue to do this each month, chances are excellent that the woman will be pregnant within a year. Indeed, the chances are about 85%. There are, however, couples who do all that they are supposed to do, and nothing happens. This is the point at which a doctor may be called upon to intervene.

The first help that a doctor gives may be no more than I have just described. He will make sure that they know how and when to have intercourse. He will teach the woman how to use the sympto-thermal method. He will tell them to try for a year without any sort of contraception. And it is still possible that conception may not occur. What then?

Either right at the beginning or at this point the doctor will wish to do some further examination and testing. The cause of the infertility may be in the husband, in the wife or in both. It may be a physical (mechanical) problem. It may be a blockage in the genital tract. It may be a hormone problem. It may be a disease, such as endometriosis. It may be a deficiency in the sperm. It may be a type of immune reaction. It may even be a cause that cannot be

212

identified — which can be one of the most difficult situations for a couple to accept.

Whatever the problem, if it is with the man it may well be easier to diagnose and easier to treat. If treatment is not possible, this may be discovered more quickly in the man than in the woman. The range of male problems is more limited and so are recognized treatments. Nevertheless, in about 35% of cases of infertility, the reason resides in the man; while in 20% it is a male problem combined with what might otherwise be a minor problem in the woman.[117]

One area of problems in the man is related to the production and maturation of sperm. This can happen for many reasons, some of which are susceptible to successful treatment. One such problem is called a varicocele. It is a condition somewhat like varicose veins, but occurring in the veins which lead away from the testicles (usually the left one). It can often be corrected by surgery and, after a recovery period of some months, sperm production increases. About 50% of these cases result in successful impregnation.[118]

In some cases sperm production is inhibited by hormone deficiencies or imbalances. Sperm production depends on a complex interrelationship of glands and hormones. There are in the human body various sorts of glands. Some of them, such as sweat glands or salivary glands, produce substances which they release through ducts. Other glands are ductless and release what they produce directly into the

---

[117] Cf. Menning, *op.cit.*, p. 59.

[118] Cf. Menning, *op.cit.*, p 61.

bloodstream. They are known as endocrine glands and it is glands such as these which produce hormones. In the case of sperm production three glands in particular are involved: the hypothalamus, the pituitary and the testicles. The hypothalamus releases a hormone which causes the pituitary to release FSH (follicle stimulating hormone) and LH (luteinizing hormone).[119] FSH acts on certain cells in the testicles to produce sperm, while LH acts on other testicular cells to produce testosterone (another hormone). When the level of testosterone is high enough, it causes the hypothalamus to signal the pituitary to slow down the LH and FSH.

Problems in producing sperm, therefore, may be treated by hormone therapy affecting the hypothalamus and pituitary relationship, or the testicles themselves — presupposing, of course, that in either case the sperm-producing tissue in the testicles is otherwise normal. One treatment involves the use of a drug called clomiphene citrate (sold under the name of Clomid or Serophene). Exactly how it works is uncertain.[120] It appears, however, that it stops the hypothalamus from detecting the rising levels of testosterone, thus allowing the pituitary to keep producing FSH and LH. This increases sperm production. Since it takes about two and a half months for sperm to be produced and come to maturity, the clomiphene will be given in small doses over several months. There are some undesirable side effects to which the doctor must be alert.

---

[119] These are the same hormones that act on the testes in the man and the ovaries in a woman.

[120] Cf. *1989 Physicians' Desk Reference*, 43rd edition, p. 2032 (hereafter referred to as *PDR*).

214

Some studies indicate improved fertility, while others are more indefinite.[121] Clomiphene seems relatively safe. It can be taken as a pill and, although it is not cheap, it does cost less than some other therapies.

Another drug, Pergonal, is composed of gonadotropins (a type of hormone) which are extracted from the urine of menopausal women. It is quite potent and can produce serious side effects, so it must be employed quite carefully. It is used together with injections of human chorionic gonadotropin (HCG: a hormone produced by the placenta), sold under the name of Profasi. This therapy is useful only in cases where there is some deficiency in the function of the hypothalamus, and such cases are rather rare. It should be used only by doctors who are expert in the treatment of infertility.[122] It is given by injection and can be very expensive.

There are also fertility problems which reside in the testicles themselves. These may result from such things as mumps, testicular damage, drug abuse, alcohol abuse, or the lack of sperm producing cells. In such circumstances there *may* be some treatment available, but in some cases nothing can be done.

In all of the cases just referred to, one part of the diagnosis will be a sperm count. This will examine the number of sperm per cubic centimeter, the ability of the sperm to move, and the percentage of irregular or malformed sperm. One moral problem that occurs here will be the way in which semen is gathered for analysis. Masturbation is not

---

[121] Cf. Menning, *op.cit.*, p. 61.

[122] Cf. *PDR*, p. 2030.

morally acceptable as a method. It is allowable, however, to make use of a type of condom called a silastic sheath. It is perforated and is used during normal intercourse. It allows initial ejaculation into the vagina and then seals itself to contain the remainder of the semen which can then be used for analysis.[123]

In a man the sperm are constantly being produced, taking about two and a half months to come to maturity. In a woman the process is quite different. Eggs form in the ovaries while she is still a child in the womb. Most of them never develop very far, but a large number remain. Once she reaches puberty, the eggs are ready to mature and, in normal situations, each month one of them, usually in alternate ovaries, ripens and is ejected from the ovary. This will continue until menopause, so that usually, in her lifetime, about 400-500 eggs are produced — as opposed to the millions of sperm always being produced by the man.

If it is the woman who has the difficulty with fertility, it may be harder to diagnose and more complicated to treat. Here, too, the problems may be merely mechanical, such as blockages in the fallopian tubes. Depending on the cause and seriousness of such conditions, treatment may range from relatively easy all the way to impossible.

Infertility may be due to a variety of abnormalities in the uterus. It may, for example, be divided into two segments by a septum of uterine tissue. This may make normal uterine expansion impossible and so a pregnancy would never come to successful conclusion. The uterus may contain scar tissue from damage of some sort or from

---

[123] Cf. Donald T. DeMarco, "Catholic Moral Teaching and TOT/GIFT" in *Reproductive Technologies, Marriage and the Church*, p. 127.

surgery. There may be fibroid tumors which are benign but which also interfere with uterine expansion or implantation. In cases such as these — or cases of tubal blockage — surgery *may* be able to correct the condition. This is especially true in view of modern methods of microsurgery or laser surgery. Both of these techniques can make tiny repairs with minimal damage to surrounding cells.

The uterus or cervix may also be damaged as the result of abortion, especially when it was performed in teenage years. The abortion industry, however, is not very willing to explain that to teenagers — and it even wants to make sure that they will never be obliged to discuss it with their parents. They make so much money that they would rather not risk losing it by offering truthful explanations of the damage for which they are responsible.

There are also other types of mechanical blocks or barriers which may occur.[124] Many of these are due to what is generically called pelvic inflammatory disease (PID). In almost every instance PID can be traced back to diseases transmitted by sexual intercourse or infections from such things as an IUD (intrauterine device). Sexual activity with multiple partners is a perfect way to end up with PID — and so to end up being infertile. The increased promiscuity of recent years has caused an enormous rise in PID, with its resultant damage to the female reproductive system. About 20 years ago blockages due to this sort of damage were responsible for about 25% of the cases of infertility in women. They now account for 50%![125]

---

[124] Cf. Menning, *op.cit.*, pp. 50-53.

[125] Cf. Menning, *op.cit.*, p. 51.

Bacterial infections (e.g., gonorrhea or chlamydia — which is now the most common venereal disease) are recurrent, damaging and even lead to death. Infection eats into the soft tissues of uterus and fallopian tubes and causes damage which quickly becomes irreversible. Each time the infection flares up it causes more harm. Among women who have only one episode of such infections, about 15% are left infertile. Of those who have three episodes, about 75% will be infertile.

It is interesting to note that chlamydia seems to be more common among women who use contraceptive pills.[126] Whether that is due to the pill or to the fact that so many pill users are promiscuous, I could not say. In any case it seems to me that our society hesitates to point all of this out, especially to the young who will be most likely to be affected by all the consequent suffering. After all, no none wants to be a party-pooper. It seems that we would prefer to let our children suffer and die rather than risk offending them by telling the truth. In any case, PID is a prevalent cause of infertility and can be impossible to correct.

Another common cause of infertility is endometriosis. This is a disease whose origin is unknown. The endometrium is the tissue which lines the uterus and which breaks down and is the source of the menstrual flow during a woman's period. When a woman has endometriosis, this tissue is found at other places in her body. It may be within the fallopian tubes, on the ovaries, on the bladder or in the peritoneal cavity. Each month, when a woman has her period, this tissue also breaks down. In its abnormal sites it causes scar tissue and blockage. It may cause

---

[126] Cf. Menning, *op,cit.*, p. 53.

adhesions and even make intercourse painful. Symptoms of pain may indicate its presence, but it cannot be diagnosed without the use of a laparoscope to see where the endometrial tissue is located. Because the scar tissue causes blockages, it may give rise to infertility by closing the tubes and preventing sperm from meeting ovum. It may also damage the ovaries themselves, causing scar tissue on the surface and thus gradually destroying the capacity of the ovary to release eggs. Some of these effects may be relieved by surgery.

It has also been noted that in many cases pregnancy seems to cure endometriosis, at least temporarily. This is probably due to the fact that during pregnancy the monthly breakdown of endometrial tissue does not occur and so the sites have time to heal. Because of this some doctors have treated the condition with medicines such as Danazol, which is a synthetic male hormone.[127] It acts on the pituitary gland so as to suppress the signals which cause production of estrogen and progesterone. It causes what is referred to as "pseudo-menopause." Ovulation and menstruation are temporarily suppressed, and the affected sites have time to heal. In mild cases it may help, but its success is never guaranteed. It has side effects which can be serious, so its use must be carefully monitored.

One of the mysteries about endometriosis is that it seems to cause infertility even in many women who have only mild cases, in which there is no apparent blockage or damage. Why this should be so, no one knows. In some ways that makes it even more difficult for the infertile couple. There seems to be no reason why conception

---

[127] Cf. Kate Weinstein, *Living with Endometriosis*, New York, pp. 81-87.

should not occur, but the fact is that it does not. There are numerous theories.[128] Painful intercourse (dyspareunia) may result in less frequent intercourse, or may prevent full penetration, or may cause muscle spasms which affect the working of the fallopian tubes. The misplaced bits of endometrial tissue produce prostaglandins (another type of hormone). These may have various effects: Slowing the motility of the sperm, decreasing or increasing muscle movement in uterus and tubes (thus leading to failure of egg and sperm to meet or rapid movement of the embryo into the uterus before it is developed enough to implant), causing uterine contractions which interfere with implantation. The misplaced endometrium also may cause an immune reaction, forming antibodies which attack the normal endometrium or the sperm. All of these, however, are conjectures. *No one really knows the cause and so no one knows the solution either.* It is, perhaps, one of the most frustrating sources of infertility.

Infertility in a woman may also stem from problems in the endocrine system, which means problems related to hormone production or balance. We saw that in the man there is a relationship between sperm production and the working of the hypothalamus, the pituitary and the testicles. In a woman there is a similar relationship between egg maturation and the working of the hypothalamus, the pituitary and the ovaries. The same hormones, FSH and LH, are responsible for quite similar effects. About half of female infertility problems can be traced to difficulties in

---

[128] *Ibid.*, pp. 126-128.

ovulation or the endocrine system.[129] A few of the ovulation problems may be due to lack of ovarian tissue as a result of chromosomal abnormalities in the woman herself or to premature ovarian failure in early adulthood. In these cases, there is nothing that can be done to correct the problem.

When anovulation (the failure to ovulate) happens at irregular intervals, it would indicate that the ovaries are functional, but there is most likely some hormonal problem. This irregularity of ovulation is a factor that the doctor should check early in the process of treating infertility. (It sometimes happens that women fail to ovulate after they have stopped using birth control pills. They may need treatment in order to resume regular ovulation).

A woman may menstruate every month even when, at times, she has not ovulated. How can she know if ovulation has occurred? The most simple way is to check her basal temperature, just as would be done in the Symptothermal method of family planning. Another way, not too difficult either, is to check the level of progesterone in the blood. If the evidence indicates that ovulation is *not* occurring every month, there is a relatively safe treatment. This is the drug called Clomid (clomiphene citrate) which was mentioned earlier. Therapy of this sort should be undertaken only after careful diagnostic evaluation by a physician experienced in this area. If ovulation has not been reestablished after treatment for three of the woman's cycles, then the use of this powerful drug should be stopped

---

[129] Cf. Menning, *op. cit.*, p. 45.

and the case revaluated.[130]   It is *not* recommended for treatment in cases where the ovaries seem to be functioning normally.

If clomiphene citrate is not successful in restoring ovulation, other therapies may be tried. Pergonal is one of the drugs which may be used.[131] It is given by injection. It contains FSH and LH, so it causes the egg follicles to mature. It does not, however, cause the eggs to burst out of the follicles once mature. Instead, an injection of HCG is given for that purpose, once the follicle is ripe (which can be seen by ultrasound). Since Pergonal, like Clomid, causes multiple ovulation, it can also lead to multiple births. With Clomid the chance of multiple pregnancy is 10%, while with Pergonal it is 20%. Again, since both Pergonal and HCG are quite potent, there must be careful diagnosis, close monitoring and very careful attention to side effects — some of which may be quite serious.

As you move up the line from clomiphene to further, more potent, drugs, you also run the risk of damage to the ovaries themselves. Cysts may form and the ovaries may become enlarged, so all of these drugs should be used with caution and only in the hands of specialists. If Clomid and Pergonal both fail to produce a pregnancy, the next step may be a drug called Metrodin. While Pergonal is composed of equal amounts of FSH and LH, Metrodin has a far greater amount of FSH and a relatively small portion of LH. Again, any use of the drugs should be preceded by careful physical examination.   As with Pergonal, the

---

[130] Cf. *PDR*, p. 2033.


[131] Cf. *PDR*. pp. 2030-2031.

222

Metrodin is given by injection to stimulate the follicles and the HCG is used to cause the eggs to break out onto the surface of the ovary. Because of the strong effect of Metrodin, the physician should examine the woman *at least every other day* during therapy and for at least two weeks afterwards. This is to spot as early as possible any signs of excessive enlargement of the ovaries.[132]

It should be noted that Clomid, Pergonal and Metrodin all cause multiple ovulation. This means that there is with all of them the possibility of multiple conceptions. Statistics indicate that Clomid's use results in multiple births about 10% of the time and both Pergonal and Metrodin more than 20% of the time. For this reason, as the physician monitors the growth of the eggs, he should warn the couple *against* intercourse if the number of eggs is excessive. Otherwise there could be so many conceptions as to make it impossible for the pregnancy to come to term. This is also why therapy should always begin with the smallest doses.

Each level of these therapies demands greater attention and, therefore, more time on the part of the physician and his staff. As a result, each level becomes increasingly expensive. Each course of treatment may involve three of the woman's cycles. As of 1988, the price *per cycle* for each was: (1) Clomid, $30-$250; (2) Pergonal, $150-$900; (3) Metrodin, $225-$1350. If a couple went through all three levels with three treatments at each level, the full price could range from $1115 to $7500. The chances of becoming pregnant — if poor ovarian function really was

---

[132] Cf. *PDR*, pp. 2020-2030.

the cause of infertility — is 30% for Clomid and 50% for Pergonal or Metrodin.[133]

This therapy is expensive and the specialist who does it must invest a great amount of time and money into it. Expensive equipment is required for diagnosis, laboratory work and monitoring of treatment. He will need a staff of people to work with him and space for offices. In view of this, the physician should be especially honest with himself about the prolonging of any of the various courses of treatment. His honest and sincere medical motivation may all too easily be influenced by financial concerns. It is also easy for a doctor to be so concerned about his patient — and, in this area especially, about their pain and frustration — that it is especially hard to admit defeat. Yet real care and concern, also demand honesty, so that people are given a chance to face reality and begin to grow from there, rather than being subject to the frustration of a constantly offered but false hope.

It would seem that none of the therapies of infertility that I have described in this chapter are of a type which should be immediately considered immoral. In each of them there are moral concerns of which we should be aware. The seriousness of side effects should be carefully weighed against the possible benefits. They should not be presented, either, as the first steps leading finally to *in vitro* fertilization or any other immoral method of dealing with infertility. It should also be noted that all of the hormone treatments can have effects on a woman's emotional life and that these effects are not in her imagination. They are real. As

---

[133] Cf. David S. McLaughlin, M.D., "A Scientific Introduction to Reproductive Technologies," *Reproductive Technologies, Marriage and the Church, Pope John Research Center*, 1988, p.56.

efforts are made to overcome infertility, the undulations of hope and disappointment are often amplified by the drugs themselves. The effect of this on the marriage should be considered.

I began by saying that a little learning is a dangerous thing. It would be dangerous for me to pretend to a medical knowledge that I do not have! For that reason especially I have tried to be most careful in all that I have said and I have made use of sources of information that offer adequate knowledge for our present purposes.

A little learning is also a danger here, in the sense that medicine knows something about the problems of infertility, but there is, in truth, even much more that remains unknown. The fact that treatment works only 30% or 50% or 10% of the time is itself a clear and obvious indication of just how much is *not* known. There is a goodly amount of knowledge combined with an enormous amount of educated guesswork. We are dealing with a complex and obscure mechanism when we get into the area of hormone therapy. Indeed, in some instances therapies are used with the frank admission that no one knows *how* they work and no one can even predict *if* they will work — except to give some percentage of their overall *chance* of success. We must admit all of this and then be respectfully cautious in what we do. And we must always be open to learn.

A couple are faced with the fact that they are infertile. They will, one would hope, get past that initial temptation of feeling guilt because "I am infertile" or anger because "you are infertile." The fact is, "*We* are infertile." They begin to look into causes and what, if anything, can be done. The man has apparently fertile sperm. The woman ovulates. They may have tried some of the therapies described in the preceding chapter. So far, nothing has worked. By this time they will have had to overcome a host of hurdles — physical, emotional and financial. What next? Does there remain something that can be done?

They will, of course, be faced with still more decisions. Various alternatives will be presented to them. At this point, however, they will have passed the stage at which the proposed treatments are most easily seen as being morally acceptable. Techniques offered from this point onward *may* still be *assisting* the couple in the natural achievement of pregnancy; most, however, will be easily recognized as *replacing* them — thus being clearly morally unacceptable. Some will obviously be no more than technical jargon or catchy acronyms used to hide one simple word — adultery.

In fact, the variety of methods offered can seem almost bewildering. Why so many? There are a few reasons. One is that the causes of infertility are so varied. Another is that the causes are simply not understood — and so all

226

sorts of efforts will be made. Still another is that the extent of infertility at the present time makes the operation of a fertility clinic a potentially booming business. It is, indeed, a very lucrative business *even if it never produces a single pregnancy*! In 1981, in Norfolk, Virginia, the first United States IVF baby was born and immediately IVF centers began to spring up all around the country. About 100 of them are now in operation, charging fees of $3000 to $7000 *per cycle* and one-third of them have not yet been able to report the birth of a single IVF baby![134]

This whole area of the technological production of babies should be looked at quite thoughtfully. There are methods offered which are obviously immoral, and so should not be used at all. Even if methods are morally acceptable, they should be carefully considered. There are widely varying rates of success and these should be closely scrutinized. Suppose, for example, that some method claims a success rate of 30%. What does that mean? If it means that 30% of the couples who tried it succeeded in having a child, that may sound encouraging. But is it? One question to ask is how many *cycles* were involved. If 100 women attempted the method and 30 became pregnant, that is 30%. But most methods do not work on the first try. If the average pregnancy took 5 cycles to accomplish, then 100 women means 500 cycles. If 30 of them succeed in having a baby, then the real percentage is 30 successes out of 500 attempts — which is only 6%.

Another obvious question ought to be whether the success rate is based on actual births or on pregnancies. In many instances certain methods have a much higher rate of

---

[134] Cf. McLaughlin, *op. cit.*, p. 58.

ectopic pregnancies.  These may be counted as pregnancies, but they will not result in births.  Even when the statistics are based on numbers of births, they may be misleading.  How many were multiple births?  And, how many were born and did not long survive?

Finally, you should know whose rates of success are being used.  Are they the real rates of *this* doctor at *this* clinic?  Or are they overall rates in the country?  Are they the rates only of certain research centers?  Are they the rates for a year?  Or a whole practice?  Or just one month that happened to be especially good?  *And remember that you pay as much for the failures as for the successes.*

There are, in other words, a multitude of preliminary questions to be considered, and things I have just mentioned do not begin to exhaust the possibilities.  However, what about the methods themselves?

One area of endeavor involves someone other than husband and wife.  No matter how we may try to explain or rationalize this, it is and always will be wrong.  It is contrary to both the unity and fidelity that are at the heart of marriage.  One such procedure is what is referred to as SET (surrogate embryo transfer).[135]  This is a method taken from cattle breeding.  Numerous eggs from a good breeding cow are fertilized and the embryos are then put into a number of other cows to implant and grow.  In 1983 the first human example of this procedure was reported.  The procedure involves an "egg donor."  A man's sperm is used to artificially inseminate a woman other than his wife.  Prior to this, his wife and the other woman are treated so as to cause their menstrual cycles to coincide, and the other

---

[135] Cf. McLaughlin, *op. cit.*, p. 60; Menning, *op.cit.*, pp. 88-89.

228

woman may also be given drugs to produce multiple ovulation. If the husband's sperm has successfully fertilized an egg or eggs, they are allowed to develop and descend into the uterus, where they will float about for a short time before beginning to implant. They are removed before implantation and put into the uterus of the wife.

It should be evident to anyone that such a procedure reduces a woman to the level of breeding stock. The child, of course, will be genetically related to the husband and the other woman, even though it is the wife goes through the pregnancy. The "donor" may be paid about $250.00 per cycle and the couple pay about $3000 per cycle.

As I said, SET was developed from cattle breeding. It is interesting to note that its commercial aspects have also been carried over into its human application.[136] An effort was made to patent the process and charge for its use, and in 1985 a group called Fertility and Genetics Research, Inc., began selling stock with the intention of franchising ovum transfer centers — by which, of course, they mean fertilized ova, which are really embryos. It's a plan similar to the way in which such companies as Pizza Hut or Dunkin Donuts might set up operations.

Another method that is simply a form of adultery is referred to as AID (artificial insemination by donor). This is also basically a cattle breeding procedure. Sperm is "donated" by means of masturbation. It may be kept frozen and is then put into a woman's genital tract during the fertile time of the month. If she becomes pregnant, of course, the child is not her husband's. The action here, as in SET, is simply another form of adultery. Of course, AID

---

[136] Cf. Menning, *op.cit.*, p. 89.

has its commercial side as well and has given rise to "sperm banks," where sperm is kept frozen until sold. It is also possible, by the way, to take eggs from a woman and insert them into another so that they can be fertilized by her husband — a process that sounds somewhat like SET, although in this case only the unfertilized eggs are transferred.

All of these procedures, as I said, violate the unity and fidelity of marriage. They are quite depersonalizing to everyone involved, and perhaps most of all to the "donors" who are, of course, expected to be never heard from again — who may, indeed, be kept anonymous in the first place.

Perhaps the most dehumanizing of all the procedures is that of "surrogate motherhood." (Isn't it annoying how we always manage to find such technical or noble sounding names for our most demeaning activities?) In this instance a woman is simply hired to become pregnant and then hand over her baby to the couple who hired her. There are actually businesses which have been set up to bring together potential parents and potential surrogates. They charge from $25,000 to $50,000 for their service and pay the surrogate a fee of perhaps $10,000.[137] Since the actual selling of a person is almost everywhere illegal, the money given to the surrogate is defined as a "fee for her services." Clean language strikes again! The semen may come from the husband who is buying the baby or from a donor. In this latter case, of course, the child is not even the offspring of his new father's adultery! There is, in fact, no physical relationship at all.

---

[137] Cf. Menning, *op.cit.*, p. 156.

In one very recent case, two women were hired as surrogates (for the usual $10,000). The couples who hired them used their own eggs and sperm, fertilized *in vitro*. Both women had babies — one, in fact, had triplets. One of the surrogates spoke of her sadness in giving up the child.[138] It astounds me to find myself living in a society which cannot see the wrongness of all of this. Instead, it is by many taken for granted that babies can be exchanged like any other commodity. Persons are turned into merchandise, and men and women into breeding stock.

I have already spoken of IVF in preceding chapters, where I explained the various moral problems involved in it, so I need not repeat it all here. I should, perhaps, indicate that what I am referring to as IVF is what is also referred to by many as IVF-ET, which means *in-vitro* fertilization with embryo transfer. It might, however, be of interest to say something about the statistics. Newspaper reports all too often encourage couples to try IVF, because they make it sound so simple and acceptable. Of course, they usually have neither the inclination nor the knowledge necessary to make a moral judgement in the matter, but neither do they generally report *all* the facts. The following sample may give you some ideas of what is involved.[139]

In a study of 296 patients undergoing IVF, some 1595 eggs were removed and 1356 of them were fertilized and transferred as embryos back into the uterus. This resulted

---

[138] Cf. *New York Times*, Sunday, August 12, 1990, p. 1A.

[139] Cf. Lorna L. Cvetkovich, M.D., "The Reproductive Technologies: A Scientific View," in *The Gift of Life*, Pope Paul VI Institute Press, Omaha, 1990, p. 9.

in 151 pregnancies. Some of these, of course, were multiple, so it does *not* mean that 151 women became pregnant. In fact, there were 17 sets of twins and one of triplets. That brings the number of women down to 132 — which still seems a tremendous percentage (44.6%). However, only 81 live births took place. Again, if we take count of twins and triplets, it would indicate that 62 of the women gave birth. That is almost 21%. We must not, however, lose sight of one vital reality. In the process 1356 human lives were begun *in vitro*. Only 151 succeeded in beginning life in the womb (that is 11%) and only 81 lived long enough to be born (that is about 6%). To produce 81 successfully delivered babies, 1275 embryos were sacrificed.

It should be noted also that *in vitro* fertilization is also performed under other names. One such is a procedure called ZIFT (zygote intrafallopian transfer). I will later refer to another procedure which is called GIFT (gamete intrafallopian transfer). It might be well to point out here one basic difference between them. A gamete is a "germ cell," that is to say, it is a sperm or an ovum. In GIFT, as we shall see, the process deals with gametes — unfertilized cells. A zygote is, on the other hand, a fertilized ovum, which is to say that it is an embryo. It is a person. It is called a zygote before it begins the process of cell division.

In ZIFT the ova are taken from the ovaries after they are stimulated to produce multiple ovulation. Semen is taken, usually by masturbation. The ova are fertilized and then put into the fallopian tube. There is no difference, in terms of moral judgement, between ZIFT and IVF. The only difference in practice is that in IVF the embryos are allowed to develop for about three days and are placed in the uterus. In fact, it is my understanding that ZIFT is really a misnomer. A zygote is only a zygote before cell division. In ZIFT there may actually be two or three cell divisions which take place before the embryo is returned to the tube. The only advantage of one over the other would seem to be that placement in the tube allows the embryo to do more of its developing within the body of its mother — which everyone agrees is the safest place for it. ZIFT is and remains, however, just another form of IVF.

In 1980 a procedure, which came to be known as LTOT (lower tubal ovum transfer), was first described by Kreitmann and Hodgen who had worked with monkeys at the National Institutes of Health. The tubes of monkeys were tied. Eggs were then taken and placed in the lower portion of the tube and the monkeys were allowed to mate. Of 31 monkeys, 5 became pregnant (16%). It seemed to be a procedure which would be of special help to women who had been infertile because of damaged tubes. The procedure was further researched in 1983 at St. Elizabeth Medical Center (a Catholic hospital) in Cincinnati by Doctors McLaughlin, Troike and Tegenkemp. One of their major concerns was to develop a procedure that would be morally acceptable within the Catholic Church.[140] The LTOT procedure, as such, does not raise a moral problem. What is moved is an egg. There is no manipulation of embryos. The couple are advised to have normal intercourse before the procedure and the day after. The procedure, in other words, is designed to help normal intercourse to become fertile. It does not in any way replace it. The

---

[140] Cf. McLaughlin, *op. cit.*, pp. 63-65.

problem was that the procedure was tried in 65 cycles with about 40 women, and none of them became pregnant.[141]

The procedure was then modified by Dr. McLaughlin and his associates. The first change was that the egg should be placed as high as possible in the tube, thus allowing more time, if it is fertilized, for it to develop on its way to the uterus. They then added a still further refinement which made a considerable change in the procedure. Along with the ovum they also inserted sperm into the tube. They now called it TOTS (tubal ovum transfer with sperm). The sperm was collected by use of a silastic sheath during normal intercourse. (This procedure was described in the preceding chapter, when I spoke of collecting sperm for analysis.) The sperm was "washed" and concentrated before being used. Washing really means separating the sperm from the seminal fluid. It is then put into another sterile liquid which will not harm it or interfere with its fertility. This is done to remove the prostaglandins, which are normally neutralized by the cervical mucus. If not removed, they could cause excess movement (peristalsis) in the fallopian tubes. The fertilized egg might then move too quickly and, therefore, be unable to implant when it reaches the uterus, since the endometrium might not be ready to receive it.

The ovum or ova were placed in a catheter and then sperm were drawn into the same catheter, separated from the egg by an air bubble. This prevented fertilization until they were all released into the upper end of the fallopian tube. Thus fertilization is *in vivo* rather than *in vitro*. This also makes the procedure more desirable from a medical

---

[141] Cf. Donald T. DeMarco, "Catholic Moral Teaching and TOT/GIFT," in *Reproductive Technologies, Marriage and the Church*, pp. 122-139.

point of view as well. There is no doubt that the mother's body is the best place for it to happen, and no one is yet sure what sorts of harm take place because of fertilization in a dish.

Before I go on to talk about the moral aspects of TOTS, I would like to say something about the procedure known as GIFT (gamete intrafallopian transfer). This was first publicized by Doctor Ricardo Asch in 1984. He had developed it at almost the same time that the team in Cincinnati were working on TOTS. The two procedures are almost identical. One obvious difference is that the team working on TOTS were intent on finding a procedure that would be in accord with Catholic morality, and so they found a way to avoid masturbation. The GIFT team had done their studies by using masturbation. You will find, in fact, that some people tend to use the terms interchangeably, and many have described GIFT as acceptable to Catholic practice. If, in fact, the sperm is gathered for GIFT in a silastic sheath during normal intercourse — as can surely be done — then the moral judgement on both would be the same.

But what is that moral judgement? Opinions are divided. Some theologians find the procedure morally acceptable and others do not. This is not by any means unusual when we try to evaluate some new process or discovery. Many people think that the Church just makes its decisions on the basis of pure authority. This is not so. Final decisions are *never* made without full and careful study — and that frequently involves stages of disagreement, even among experts. That is, in fact, one of the clearest signs that the teaching of the Church comes from a living Spirit and not a dead letter.

Why do they disagree? The reason is easy enough to understand. I mentioned earlier that some methods of overcoming infertility are obviously ways of assisting the natural process; and this is a first clue that they *may* be morally acceptable. Other methods are clearly separated from the natural process and replace it; and this is an immediate and certain indication that they are wrong. In TOTS/GIFT some theologians see an assistance to the natural process and others see a replacement. If you stop and think about it, I am sure that you will realize that there is no clear and immediate answer to it, at least not right now.

All of them, of course, begin by looking to see if there is anything clearly and obviously wrong. Does fertilization take place outside the body? For both TOTS and GIFT, the answer is no. Are any eggs fertilized and then discarded? Again, no. Is the semen gathered in a wrong way, such as by masturbation? For TOTS (if used in its original proto- col) the answer is again, no. For GIFT as used by some doctors, the answer is yes. In those instances GIFT would be wrong. But if the doctor using GIFT is willing to make use of a silastic sheath during normal intercourse, then the answer here, too, is no. Does the process involve true marital intercourse? For TOTS, yes. For GIFT, yes, if done as I have described. So far they both look good, and there should, one would think, be no reason for disagreement. But there is, and it is a very real reason.

The sperm and egg are removed from the body, manipu- lated to some degree and then put back into the upper end of the tube, just about a half inch inside the fimbriated (fringed) end. A number of very good and reputable theologians see this as a form of artificial insemination, separated in time and place from the act of intercourse itself. (Intercourse takes place at home, before the proce-

236

dure begins, and the operation will be done a few hours later.) The procedure does not simply clear the way for the sperm and ovum to meet in the normal course of events. Instead, it intervenes in the process and in some way changes things. Therefore they would consider it wrong. It *replaces* the normal process.

Other theologians see the procedure as a means of *assisting* rather than replacing. It is viewed as bringing the sperm, ejaculated in normal marital intercourse, to the place where it is intended to be. The procedure of washing simply does what the woman's body would have done normally. The eggs are also moved, because one of the problems in many cases of infertility is in the fact that the eggs remain on the surface of the ovary and are not drawn into the tube as they should be. The procedure, therefore, is seen as assistance.

What does the official teaching of the Church have to say about it? So far, nothing. That, of course, is not unusual. Those who exercise the teaching authority of the Church have no desire to mislead people, and will not attempt to give official approval or disapproval when a matter is unclear or disputed among reputable theologians.[142]

Where does this leave couples who are trying to decide if they can morally use TOTS/GIFT? Well, both sides have strong and valid reasons for what they say. Both sides are held by good and reputable experts. There has been no final statement by Church authority — there has, in fact, been no statement at all about TOTS/GIFT. In such a case it is

---

[142] For a good discussion of both sides of the question, I would suggest that you read the articles by David S. McLaughlin, John M. Haas, William E. May, Donald T. De Marco and Donald G. McCarthy in *Reproductive Technologies, Marriage and the Church*.

perfectly allowable to look at the reasons on both sides and come to your own honest conclusion. You must take the guidelines that are available and make a decision. It should not be done lightly. *I am not saying* that in every case of disagreement among theologians everything is up for grabs. *I am saying* that (1) when *reputable* theologians disagree, and (2) both sides present arguments that seem strong and probable, and (3) the weight of *official* Church teaching does not clearly support one side or the other, then you may feel morally justified in choosing either alternative, depending on how you see the strength of the arguments.

The success rate of TOTS/GIFT has been good. The pregnancy rate has been about 30% as compared to the overall 10% for IVF. (It should be noted, however, that the most successful IVF clinics claim a rate of 15% to 20%.)[143] GIFT's highest rates have been in cases of endometriosis (32%) and unexplained infertility (31%). Note, however, that all of these percentages — IVF and GIFT — are pregnancy rates and about one-third of them failed to produce a live birth.

By the way, there is one more thing that I should explain a bit further, and that is the use of the silastic sheath that I have referred to so often. You may think that gathering the sperm in this way is just one of those "Catholic things." Not so. Even in gathering sperm for analysis this is better in a medical perspective than is masturbation. Experts who have studied its use have come to the conclusion — on purely medical grounds — that it is better for both semen analysis and for help with fertility. The first reason is the material of which it is made. It is chemically neutral and

---

[143] Cf. Cvetkovich, *op.cit.*, pp. 12-13.

238

therefore does less harm to the sperm than is done by a glass jar or the ordinary latex condom. Secondly, the ejaculation differs. It is improved by the stimulation of the female in intercourse and is therefore a better sample than one obtained by masturbation — and, therefore, probably more fertile.[144]

In an earlier chapter I spoke of testimony given by Doctor Jerome Lejeune in the Tennessee frozen embryo case. In that same testimony Doctor Lejeune also made some interesting statements about our present methods of attempting to treat infertility. Much of our effort now seems to go into the mechanics of getting egg and sperm together so as to produce conception. In some cases, such as damaged tubes, that may continue to be the problem. There are, however, many cases in which infertility remains unexplained. Even in the case of endometriosis, where the system seems to function but pregnancy does not occur, it is not enough to say that it is due to the endometriosis, because we do not know *why*. Doctor Lejeune makes the significant point that our preoccupation with mechanics may be taking us on a totally false course. He sees the real answers as being in the areas of tubal repair, antibiotics and chemical factors. All of these, of course, would surely be in the realm of things done so as to make the natural process possible. Present methods, such as IVF, are quite crude efforts to mimic nature and their highest success rates are still not comparable to their enormous failure rate.

---

[144] Cf. De Marco, *op.cit.*, based on Cy Schoenfeld, *et al.*, "Evaluation of a New Silastic Seminal Fluid Collection Device," *Fertility and Sterility*, Vol. 30, No. 3, Sept., 1978, pp. 319-321; and Panayiotis M. Zavos. "Characteristics of human ejaculates collected via masturbation and a new Silastic seminal collection device," *ibid.*, Vol. 43, No. 3, March, 1985. pp 491-2.

Perhaps our time and resources should be diverted back to where they would ultimately do the most good.

One simple question — "What next?" — has generated a far from simple response. Decisions are not easy. Learn about every method that is proposed to you, if you are trying to deal with infertility. *Never* act in ignorance. This area is too important for that. It is the most sacred, most creative aspect of the marital bond in terms of its physical expression. Respect yourselves, your bodies, your sexuality. Don't allow anyone to reduce something so sacred as the start of life to a laboratory technology. It is too precious.

# CHAPTER 31

## LOVE AND PAIN

The course of true love never runs smooth. How often have you heard that or even said it yourself? It has been the basic theme of hundreds of plays, films and novels. It has been at the heart of drama, tragedy and comedy. It is a concept first put into words by Shakespeare, when Lysander says to Hermia:

Ay me! for aught that I could ever read,

Could ever hear by tale or history,

The course of true love never did run smooth...[145]

The obvious question, of course, is, "Why not?" What should run smoother than true love? After all, seventeen centuries before Shakespeare made his pronouncement, the Roman poet, Virgil, said: "Love conquers all things."[146] Why then should there ever be a hill or a valley or even a bump in its path? Who is right? If I may presume to intervene in an apparent disagreement between Shakespeare and Virgil, I would say that, in fact, both are right.

---

[145] William Shakespeare, *A Midsummer's Night's Dream*, Act I, Scene 1, lines 132-134.

[146] Virgil [Publius Vergilius Maro], *Eclogues*, X, 69.

All real love — at least in this life — seems to involve pain of some sort. How many people love someone who does not love them in return? And so their love is always filled with longing; but longing means unfulfillment, and so pain. How many parents love their children and yet are helpless to assist them when they get involved in things that will in the end destroy them? The love is real and so, too, is the pain. How many married couples start life together knowing that they are in love, only to find that being "in love" is just the beginning? To learn to live in love together is to find that you and your beloved are both weak human beings, prone to faults and sin. How very much we must grow and change before "being in love" becomes real love! But there, perhaps, is the heart of the matter. We must grow.

Even true love cannot be smooth when the lovers are full of rough edges. Love involves coming closer — in marriage, indeed, becoming *one* — and closeness of rough edges means friction. How do two porcupines make love? Very carefully. And even when we are not as bristly as porcupines, we need to take care. We need to learn not to let our rough edges damage the other's tender spots. We need to learn to love, and that means learning about yourself and about those you love. It also means mistakes along the way. It means the humility of accepting our own failures and expressing our sorrow for them; and it means the generosity of forgiving the faults of those we love. In the movie, *Love Story*, one of the characters spoke that immortal line: "Love means never having to say you're sorry." Nothing could be further from the truth. Without real repentance for our own foolish faults, love would not be possible at all.

The old romantic novels of an earlier age had their own conventions for portraying love. The lover's heart would

242

beat wildly, the cheeks would flush, the eyes would open wide, the breath would come in gasps... Symptoms of being in love? Not really. Actually they might be signs of high blood pressure or just an extra spurt of adrenalin. We're really no better at portraying it now. Perhaps we are worse. In modern novels and drama love is all too often confused with lust. Physical desire is the cheap substitute for true love. Desires are satisfied or not and then soon forgotten, only to be replaced by some new fancy. Love lasts even when desire ebbs, and the two — even though they *may* accompany each other — are never truly the same thing.

Desire and "being in love" just seem to happen with a certain spontaneity — even when in fact unwanted. Real love *never* just happens. It must be *chosen* and *fostered* and *stand the test of time*. People speak of falling in and out of love as though it were an accident, and all beyond our control. The fact is that spontaneous emotions and desires (which are all temporary) are, to some extent, out of our control. Love (which can choose to be permanent) is not.

One of the first things that must be learned about real love is that it must be freely chosen. It never comes about by chance. To love is to commit yourself and your life to another. It is to receive into your hands and heart the life of someone else.

There is probably no better example of love than the commitment made in a marriage. Marriage does not mean that you decide to live together because you happen to "be in love." Marriage is a contract, a covenant, a freely chosen commitment. It is a permanent union entered into by the most solemn vows. It is a commitment to *love* "for better or for worse, for richer or for poorer, in sickness and in health until death." It is a promise made before God and His people, the Church.

True love never does run smooth, because we are human. But if we choose to commit ourselves to love and live that commitment, then love does indeed conquer all things. It far surpasses any temporary emotion. It gently rubs away any rough edges. It grows and deepens and creates something new. The loving couple give life to each other and they begin to long also for their love to be so creative that it gives new life to a child. This is one of the characteristics of real love: It seeks to extend itself, to give life, to create. It is a quality we inherit from our Father in Heaven.

"On the part of the spouses, the desire for a child is natural: It expresses the vocation to fatherhood and motherhood inscribed in conjugal love."[147] There are, of course, many possible reasons for wanting to have a child. Some of them can be quite selfish. There are parents who have children and treat them almost as toys, wanting to love and be loved on demand and then pushing them away when they are inconvenient. There are sad cases of single women purposely becoming pregnant in order to satisfy their own longing for a child, while depriving that same child of the fuller love that ought to come from having both father and mother. There are those who see children as a way to support their image of their own manhood or womanhood. There are those who want to have an heir. There are even those who want to have the standard 2.6 children deemed necessary for their own social status. Not all children, even in marriage, come from a real depth of true conjugal love.

None of the reasons I have just mentioned is a good

---

[147] *Instruction*, n. 93.

reason for having a child. In each of these instances the child is being used. It is not desired in and for itself, to be loved and cherished. Rather it is intended to fulfill some self-centered need in the parents. There are even those who will go to great lengths to have one or two children and will then go to even greater lengths, even to the point of abortion, to prevent having any more. That bespeaks a contradiction — perhaps a generous impulse overcome, in the end, by human selfishness. It bespeaks also an attitude far removed from faith. It is an outlook so filled with a vision of autonomy that it leaves no room for God and takes control even of life and death.

Then there are those who do love and do try to grow. They long for the fulfillment of their vocation to fatherhood and motherhood — and nothing happens. They are, for whatever reason, infertile. They have a love that they share with each other and they are filled with the desire to share that mutual love with a child — and they cannot have a child of their own. There is great love and great pain. And whenever you find that mixture of love and pain, there is the potential for growth (indeed, for holiness) or for rejection.

The first reaction for many good couples in such a situation may be sorrow or anger — both of which represent pain. A deep desire is thwarted, and they feel deeply hurt. Of course, they may feel renewed hope once they decide to seek help; but, if the help goes on for months without result, the hurt becomes even deeper. I already spoke earlier of the ease with which such a couple — even with the best of intentions — can be drawn into a process which leads them to try to use means of treatment that should never be used — those means which deal death more than life or violate the most sacred aspects of their marriage.[148]  I would like to speak now of something more positive.  Their choice to do what can morally be done and to go no further is a choice which can deepen their love of each other.  It is also a choice which expresses, in actions as well as in words, the depth of their respect for the very life which they would so love to give.

Our society so often treats children as a curse.  There are couples who do all that they can in order to avoid having children.  For many, birth control is taken for granted. Children interfere with freedom.  They are an unwelcome responsibility.  They cost money and get in the way of the acquisition of things that a couple want to have.  These are attitudes that, in the end, undermine love because they reinforce the rejection of generosity.  The couple who view having children in this way are not likely to have a happy marriage.  If they cannot be generous together, they will not be generous with each other either.  They may have abundant property.  Inside they will shrivel up and die.  In the midst of all that they have, they are to be pitied.  They do not grasp the meaning of love.  They reject the true value of their own sexuality.  They are offered the gift of creating life and they turn it down.

How different are the couples who generously open their love to the gift of life.  If they are truly eager to give life, then they are all the more likely to want to give life to each other as well.  Their growth in love will not be without struggle; they are, after all, human. Each moment of struggle, however, is also an opportunity to change and to grow.  As they change, it will become all the more evident that their love is a gift.  It is freely given and freely

---

[148] Cf. *supra*, chapters 7 and 30.

246

received. You are never the owner of the one you love and you are never owned by the one who loves you. Instead, love sets you free and you choose, even more freely, to deepen and live to the end the commitment which was made on the day of marriage. The right that each one has over the other is not a right of proprietorship, but a right that comes from a freely given gift — a gift offered every day until death.

In the begetting of a child, what rights are involved? Just as husband and wife can never own each other, so they can never *own* a child. There is no right to a child in the way in which one might have a right to a piece of property. "A true and proper right to a child would be contrary to a child's dignity and character. The child is not an object to which one has a right, nor can he be considered as an object of ownership: rather, a child is a gift, 'the supreme gift' and the most gratuitous gift of marriage, and is a living testimony of the mutual giving of his parents."[149] As husband and wife, the couple confer upon each other the right to perform those natural actions which lead to the begetting of a child. This is not the same as having a right to a child.

This may be terribly hard for a couple to accept. Their intention, at first, may be truly the generous and loving desire to be parents and to give and nourish the gift of life. The temptation later may be to attempt to have a child at *any cost*. The methods proposed to them may involve enormous cost — and I am not referring here only to money. The cost may be the creation of a number of new lives and the discarding of the majority in favor of the one

---

[149] *Instruction*, n. 94.

most likely to survive. It may be the purchase of a child to be taken away from its real mother by contract. It may be infidelity to the marriage bond itself. It may be the reduction of husband and wife to mere "manufacturers" of a baby by separating the whole process from their own loving act of intercourse. All of these are costs that they would, at first, never even have considered. They may even, at the beginning have found such ideas repugnant. But the pain of the inability to have a child may make them more and more blind to the costs.

What the Church teaches is so often treated as mere rules and regulations. It is ridiculed in the press and even thrown into doubt by some theologians. It is denounced as old fashioned and too traditional. It is seen as bound up in principle and not enough interested in producing results. It is called restrictive and reactionary. And, yet, what is at the heart of all that the Church teaches? It is this: Every human being has a God-given value that should never be denied or violated by anyone. Every human being, from the moment of conception to the moment of death, is and must be treated as a child of God created to pass through this life on the way to eternal life with the Father. Every human being is loved by God and so must be loved by us. In all that the Church teaches about our power to create new human life it is simply telling us that we must never lose sight of who and what we are. We cannot claim that our goal is good and then violate the meaning of love in order to achieve it.

The couple who experience the pain of infertility must not allow that pain to make them blind to what is truly right and good. No matter how deep is their longing for a child, they must never lose sight of the fact that their value in themselves and for each other is not based on the capacity to have a child.

248

They may go through the pain of feeling guilt at what they cannot do, and yet they cannot be truly guilty in a matter beyond their control. It might help them to realize that this "guilt" probably comes from the sense of loss in the fact that they cannot give each other what they so much want. It is the feeling that comes from not being able to do all that you want to do for the one you love. In that sense it is the kind of pain that can make love grow. They can begin to say to each other, "It is *you* I love and not just what you can do for me."

They may feel anger at themselves and even at each other. Frustration produces anger, and they should not be surprised to experience it. But even this pain can make their love grow. They must begin to realize that it is not "I" who cannot have a child. It is "we" who are unable. This can bring them more fully to realize that they have come together in marriage to love each other and to share *together* whatever is painful to either. As they learn to sustain and support each other even in this trial, their love will grow.

Husband and wife have toward each other an obligation that many people hardly ever think about. It is the awesome obligation to assist in making each other holy. If I *truly* love someone, then I want that person to be happy not only here and now, but forever. I want the one I love to be all that he or she was ever meant to be. When husband and wife love in this way, then each must care about the moral goodness and immortal life of the other. This is why each must help and support the other in doing what is right and turning away from whatever is wrong and, being wrong, is destructive. No morally wrong answer to infertility can be accepted, because it means achieving a goal at the expense of doing moral damage to the one you love most of all, the one who has become one with yourself. To accept this may also seem painful, but it is again the kind of pain which leads to deeper love.

I have spoken of pain and of love, but I do not wish to leave you with the impression that pain is a good in itself. It is not. Even though there are some who seem to romanticize it, it is still pain and it hurts. What I am really saying is this: Growth in love, like most growth, has its painful aspects. Much of the pain comes from the fact that growing in love takes us outside ourselves and cuts away all that is selfish or self-centered. It demands full self-giving and the full acceptance of reality. Not all of our desires — not even the most cherished of them — will necessarily be fulfilled. This we must face, and when we can face it with the loving support of someone who cares totally for us, then unfulfilled desires and loving reality can merge into honest acceptance. Acceptance also means not focussing our minds and hearts so much on what we cannot have, that we fail to see the gifts and the love that we do have.

What advice can I give to couples who want to have children and cannot? First of all, I would say that you should look at each other and look beyond what you cannot do to what you can do. Look at your love for each other and do all that you can to make it grow. Be gentle and kind to each other. See your life together in its fullness, including God's love which has brought you together in order to love each other. Pray together and for each other. Look at those around you and let your love reach out to them. In all that you learn together, you have a great gift to give to others. Cherish that gift and share it. Don't focus on desire and end up missing reality.

The *Instruction on Procreation* says that couples who are unable to have children "must not forget that 'even when procreation is not possible, conjugal life does not for this reason lose its value. Physical sterility in fact can be for spouses the occasion of other important services to the life of the human person, for example, adoption, various forms of education works, and assistance to other families and to poor and handicapped children.'"[150] In other words, all of the love that husband and wife can share, can also reach out beyond themselves even when they do not have children of their own. That may, at first, seem a poor substitute for what they desire most of all. It can, in fact, be deeply fulfilling. The heart of this advice is this: Don't close in on yourselves. Let your love grow and allow it to be creative and productive. You will find yourselves not only loving but also deeply loved.

One final word about adoption. This is an alternative that should surely be considered. The safest way, even though there may be a long waiting period, is through a recognized adoption agency, such as those conducted by a Catholic Social Agency. I say "safest" in the sense that you are assured that the adoption is done legally and with far less risk of the birth parents reclaiming the baby and causing even greater sadness. Although the adopted child is not the physical offspring of the adopting parents, they are still — in a very real sense — its procreators. The physical bearing of the child, as wonderful as it is, is still just the first part of procreation. It is, indeed, the long years of nurturing that procreate the child into its physical and spiritual maturity. It is the same generosity and desire to create new life which inspire the adoptive parents. In fact, by the time of adoption the new parents bring with them

---

[150] *Instruction*, n. 95.

the depth of love that has grown throughout their whole struggle with infertility. If they have indeed dealt with the pain and learned the lessons it can teach, they will be a loving couple with an abundance of gifts — gifts which will enable them to offer their child a human expression of what God's creative love is all about.

No one in his right mind goes out looking for pain. But it comes along all by itself to every one of us. Love that starts out all bubbly with the heat of infatuation can, through all the struggles that are part of life, become the quiet and abiding love of maturity. It can last quietly in this life and be enjoyed for all eternity.

All love at first, like generous wine,
Ferments and frets until 'tis fine;
But when 'tis settled on the lee,
And from th'impurer matter free,
Becomes the richer still the older,
And proves the pleasanter the colder.[151]

---

[151] Samuel Butler (1612-1680), *Miscellaneous Thoughts*.

## CHAPTER 32

## HAVE SOME FUDGE

In 1832, in the process of exercising his right to veto a bill passed by congress, President Andrew Jackson said:

There are no necessary evils in government. Its evils exist only in its abuses. If it would confine itself to equal protection, and as Heaven does its rains, shower its favors alike on the high and the low, the rich and the poor, it would be an unqualified blessing.[152]

This presents a high ideal for government. Equal protection of *all* under the law is a goal to be hoped for. I suppose that if every legislator, judge and executive were perfect, then it would be a reality. Alas, both the governed and the governing are all imperfect human beings. They all have their own axes to grind and they will always be tempted to use those axes on each other when it comes to carving out the niche for protection of their own "rights" as opposed to those of others. Of course, there may be room for honest disagreement at times about just who is in the right, and that leads to debate (with or without the axes) and resolution or, at least, compromise. This may happen even on issues that seem vital and essential, and there may be true differences of conscience as well as of opinion.

---

[152] Andrew Jackson, *Veto of the Bank Bill*, July 10, 1832.

The elected official is one of those whose position may seem the most precarious. Not only does he have a conscience of his own, but he also represents a constituency formed of any number of people with any number of positions in opinion and in conscience. It is by them that he is elected and to them that he must answer — at least when he comes up for reelection. How does he reconcile himself to the fact that he represents a group which may include people whose ideas of basic moral right and wrong differ from or are even in conflict with his own? The problem is made all the more complex by reason of the fact that the one who runs for office must count on pleasing the majority of the people, if he intends to stay in office. It sounds like an almost impossible balancing act, and one would expect that it would make most officials quite happy to get out of office. Yet, as Voltaire said, "The pleasure of governing must certainly be exquisite, if we may judge from the vast numbers who are eager to be concerned with it."[153]

One of the problems that every person must face — and the politician is no exception — is just how far it is possible to compromise before reaching the point at which one violates his own conscience. Once a person passes that boundary, he begins to tear himself down. For the politician this is a very acute problem. It may seem to him that he must find a way to compromise on every issue, no matter how important, and that in this lies the way to political success and the attainment of an office in which, finally, he "can do some good." The problem, however, is that a man such as this should not be in office at all. How

<hr />

[153] Voltaire (Francois Marie Arouet), "Government," *Philosophical Dictionary*, 1764.

much faith can you put in a man who does not even follow his own conscience? Of course there are matters of policy in which people may agree on the results to be obtained and yet disagree on just how to attain them. In that instance compromise may not be wrong at all, and both the end and the means turn out to be good; but there are other cases in which this is not true.

If the politician is to be honest to himself and to his constituents — and that is essential if he is even to be worth electing to office — then he must tell them what he believes in conscience and he must live it both privately and publicly. If this costs him the election, then so be it. This is a hard choice, but *it is the only right choice.* If he attempts to do otherwise, he soon finds that he has no conscience left. "Conscience is thoroughly well-bred and soon leaves off talking to those who do not wish to hear it."[154]

The bitter loss of conscience may, for a time, be sweetened with a bit of fudge, and, as we know all too well, fudging the issues is an art in which many politicians excel. In our society we are constantly being served whole trays of fudge on governmental stands in relation to questions of "reproductive rights." Yet there can be no doubt that these questions are matters of conscience, and that they are of essential interest to both Church and civil society.

The *Instruction on Procreation* says, "The inviolable right to life of every innocent human individual and the rights of the family and of the institution of marriage constitute fundamental moral values, because they concern the natural condition and integral vocation of the human person; at the

---

[154] Samuel Butler (d. 1902), *Note-Books*, 1912.

same time they are constitutive elements of civil society and its order."[155] The topics mentioned here are so fundamental, so basic, that there is little room, if any, for compromise.

Failure to protect such rights is the beginning of the end for any society. Once any society denies the basic right to life to any category of persons within it, it sets the precedent that it can equally well choose to deny those same rights to any other group. This is precisely what happened in Nazi Germany when all rights were denied to Jews, gypsies, homosexuals, the insane and anyone else who could, for one reason or another, be declared less than human. This made every atrocity against them perfectly legal. It is also what happened in the United States when our own Supreme Court decided that slaves deserved no protection before the law. They were less than human. It is what happened in our own time when again the Supreme Court decided that the right to life for the unborn could be negated. They were no longer human. It is the same direction in which many would like to proceed in reference to the aged, the retarded, the deformed, the comatose, the disabled newborn and anyone else who does not meet their standard for "full" human life.

The person who is elected to public office in this country must now face a problem of conscience that deals with the most basic values of life itself. Legislation is being formulated in all of the areas that I mentioned at the end of the last paragraph, and everyone of those areas either is now or will become a matter of great public interest. The person who runs for office will have to face the fact that

---

[155] *Instruction*, n. 97.

256

his election may well depend on his position on matters of life and death. What does the candidate do if popular opinion runs contrary to the true voice of conscience?

For the moment I would like to limit my discussion of this area to the question as it affects the Catholic candidate or Catholic office holder. My reason is that the problem for the Catholic is quite clearly defined. The Catholic Church has a clearly defined hierarchical structure and teaching authority. As a result, its moral positions are stated clearly and publicly; and in such basic issues the candidate or office holder can have little or no doubt about what such teachings are. (Of course, the same or similar problems of conscience will exist for any other candidate — Catholic or not — when he finds himself having to frame or interpret civil laws which run contrary to the truth.)

I am also going to limit my discussion to the question of abortion and the laws related to it. I do this because the question is so clearly before us at the present time and because this issue has become a bone of contention in elections throughout the United States. The principles that I will deal with, however, will apply equally well to all of the areas mentioned above. I am also presupposing all of the information that was presented earlier in this book in regard to the origin of human life and human person.[156]

For the most part it seems that candidates and civil office holders, especially when seeking election, try to avoid limiting discussion to one single issue (unless, of course, they think that the one single issue will win the election for them). I am certainly not criticizing them if, indeed, they

---

[156] Cf. especially chapters 8-13.

do want to discuss all, or at least many, of the current issues. The problem is that, with all too many candidates, a matter of life and death such as the abortion issue, can get sidestepped, clouded over, or purposely fudged. It is a rare candidate who tries to tell the public not only what his position is, but how and why he has come to hold it. It is a rare bird, indeed, who would try to do so on a really hot issue.

In 1984 Governor Mario M. Cuomo of New York proved himself to be one of those rarest of birds. On September 13, of that year, at the University of Notre Dame, he delivered a paper entitled, "Religious Belief and Public Morality: A Catholic Governor's Perspective."[157] His position is basically this: A Catholic public official can, in good conscience, be personally and conscientiously opposed to abortion, and yet be able to vote in favor of legislation which provides funding for the performance of abortions.

The paper is, at the time of this writing, six years old, and so one might wonder why I am even bothering to respond to it. First of all, it still remains the one coherent effort by a politician to give a clear and cogent statement on the topic. For this reason it deserves our attention. Secondly, the Governor himself has not treated the paper as a matter of past history. He has, in fact, referred back to it frequently as a source of justification for later actions and statements. Thirdly, it represents a position easily adopted by

---

[157] Mario M. Cuomo, "Religious Belief and Public Morality: A Catholic Governor's Perspective," a paper prepared for delivery to the Department of Theology at the University of Notre Dame September 13, 1984. Hereafter cited as "Cuomo, *op.cit.*," with page references to the embargoed copy given to the press.

258

other public officials, and so deserves a response lest they be misled by it.

In the paragraphs which follow, I am not in any way attempting to attack Governor Cuomo personally, nor do I want to imply that he is, or that I consider him to be, dishonest in his arguments. But I am fully convinced that he is dead wrong in the position he described and supports, and that his arguments are filled with serious flaws. Near the end of his presentation he says: "I hope that this public attempt to describe the problems as I understand them, will give impetus to the dialogue in the Catholic community and beyond, a dialogue which could show me a better wisdom than I've been able to find so far."[158] It is in the spirit of that dialogue that I now write.

The Governor makes clear the fact he is and views himself as a Catholic and that "to be a Catholic is to say 'I believe' to the essential core of dogmas that distinguishes our faith."[159] We live, however, in a pluralistic society and the Catholic who holds public office "bears special responsibility. He or she undertakes to help create conditions under which *all* can live with a maximum of dignity and with a reasonable degree of freedom; where everyone who chooses may hold beliefs different from specifically Catholic ones — sometimes contradictory to them..."[160] When Catholic officials assume public office, they take an oath to preserve the Constitution which guarantees this

---

[158] Cuomo, *op. cit.*, p. 18.

[159] Cuomo, *op. cit.*, p. 4.

[160] Cuomo, *op. cit.*, p. 4.

freedom. In fact, to assure our own freedom, we must allow others the same freedom. "We know that the price of seeking to force our beliefs on others is that they might someday force theirs on us."[161]

The Governor also points out that the constitutional amendment which forbids the establishment of a State Church also "affirms my legal right to argue that my religious belief would serve well as an article of our universal public morality."[162] This is, indeed, a significant point. It means that when one is elected to public office he still has this same right and can and should still be allowed to attempt to convince others of the rightness of his position. "And surely, I can, if so inclined, demand some kind of law against abortion not because my Bishops say it is wrong but because I think that the whole community, regardless of its religious beliefs, should agree on the importance of protecting life — including life in the womb, which is at the very least potentially human and should not be extinguished casually."[163] Finally, he says, "I accept the Church's teaching on abortion. Must I insist you do? By law? By denying you Medicaid funding? By a constitutional amendment? If so, which one? Would that be the best way to avoid abortions or to prevent them?"[164]

---

[161] Cuomo, *op. cit.*, p. 5.

[162] Cuomo, *op. cit.*, p. 5.

[163] Cuomo, *op. cit.*, p. 5.

[164] Cuomo, *op. cit.*, p. 5.

260

The preceding paragraphs are a summary of the Governor's presentation of *the questions* which need to be addressed. The most basic flaws in his position are already evident in the way in which the questions themselves are being stated. He reduces the whole question to one of religious beliefs versus religious freedom. Clearly *this is not the case.* The basis for the Church's claim that abortion is wrong is not simply a matter of a "specifically Catholic" belief. It should be evident to any reader of this book that my own reasons for accepting the wrongness of abortion are not reasons founded in a specifically Catholic position. They are based on the evidence of science, which leaves no doubt that the fertilized ovum is new life, individual life, human life. There is no doubt or question of its humanity. Is the embryo a person? I would say that it is, and I have already given my arguments in earlier chapters.

Those who support abortion differ in their views. Some say that the embryo is a person, but that the woman's right to kill it takes precedence over its right to life. However, even the judges who made the *Roe v. Wade* decision would not have accepted that. In fact, in the hearing of the case one of the Justices said that the acceptance of such a position should then lead logically to the legal acceptance of the killing of a husband because he was in some way a threat to his wife's health.[165] Instead they made their ruling on the grounds that the fetus was not a person. Their position, however might not mean quite what you would expect. *Their ruling had nothing to do with the humanity or real personhood of the fetus.* It was based, instead, on the fact that the fetus, even if a *real* person, was not a *legal*

---

[165] Cf. Supreme Court, *Roe v. Wade*, arguments in No. 70-18, official transcript, pp. 27-28.

person (i.e., a citizen with rights to be preserved), because the Fourteenth Amendment extended such rights only to those who are *born* or naturalized as citizens.[166] It was a decision based on the rankest sort of legalism. Mrs. Sarah R. Weddington, the lawyer for "Jane Roe" argued, in fact, that a law which accepted the rights of the fetus was merely a statutory and not a constitutional protection (since a citizen must be *born*). In her words, "you do not balance constitutional rights of one person against mere statutory rights of another." Even she seems to speak of both as persons, but not both as citizens!

There are others who support abortion on the ground that a fetus is *not* a person. (They are not using this to mean only *legal* person.) Their argument, however, has to go against every shred of observable scientific evidence, as I have already shown in earlier chapters.

In other words, the real question is at heart not a matter of religious belief, but of evidence observable and producible by scientific procedure, from which the inference of personhood follows immediately. Acting in favor of abortion is to act contrary to science and reason. For the Catholic it also happens to mean acting against his Church as well. In other words, the Church's position can hardly be characterized as a demand of an act of blind faith in a dogmatic position. Rather, it is the exercise of the Church's authority in full support of what one can see as the truth even without an act of faith.[167] It is a question

---

[166] Cf. *Idem*, pp. 7, 24, 39.

[167] Cf. Sacred Congregation for the Doctrine of the Faith, *Declaration on Procured Abortion*, nn. 5-18.

of truth versus error, not of Church versus state. It is also a question of truth versus legalism in its worst form. To say differently is to fudge. I am *not* saying that Governor Cuomo has made his statement of the questions in bad faith. I am, however, saying that his line of thought is going to be totally colored by a basic error in the questions being asked. Even though unintentional, this is till fudging — and fudge is fudge, whether it has real sugar or just artificial sweetener.

To live in a pluralistic society does *not* mean that we have to hold back from stating and supporting what is true. Even if the abortion issue were completely a matter of religious belief (*and it is not*), we would have every right to attempt to persuade others to accept and see the truth of our position. And I mean *persuade*, not coerce or impose upon. Persuasion, however, will never occur if we say one thing and do another. In the last century slaveowners who argued against slavery could hardly have been very convincing. In Nazi Germany in the 1940's a legislator who argued against killing Jews, while still voting funding for crematoria, could hardly have been a powerful voice for truth. So it is now. To fund abortions while saying they are wrong is like warning a diabetic of the danger of sugar and then offering him a full diet of fudge. Real pluralism means the freedom to *state and live* what I believe, and to do otherwise is to mislead. In fact, when it comes to *forcing* our beliefs on others, the pro-abortion people have done that already. It is certainly a prime example of coercion to be forced, under penalty of law, to pay taxes which legislators are going to use to pay for abortions which both faith and reason tell me are immoral. It coerces me into acting against my conscience.

I am of the opinion, as is Governor Cuomo, that the passing of laws against abortion is not a final answer. What needs to change is much more than legal structure. There is a need for change in minds and hearts. But this does *not* mean that a change in law is therefore negligible. It will not come about without a change in the outlook of the majority — but isn't that what persuasion is all about? And I emphasize once more, I will never truly persuade anyone if I say one thing and do another.

What of personal freedom? What of the "right to privacy"? Even though no such right is specifically mentioned in the Constitution, the courts have construed it as being implied, especially in the Ninth Amendment, which says: "The enumeration in the Constitution, of certain rights, shall not be construed to deny or disparage others retained by the people." The implied "right to privacy" would mean that the State cannot intervene in the life of the individual in areas which are that person's business and should not be the concern of the State. Of course, there are some clear and obvious limits to that right insofar as it interferes with the legitimate rights of others. If I steal or murder, then I cannot claim that it was simply my own business and the State should stay out of it. In abortion, however, precisely that claim is being made. It is the woman's right to decide if she shall or shall not end her pregnancy by killing her child. It is justified on the grounds that the Fourteenth Amendment does not recognize her child as a person with constitutional rights. *If ever a legal situation demanded change, this is it!*

Governor Cuomo, as you would expect, does not merely ask some questions. He also offers answers. His first set of responses[168] centers on the notion that "the values derived from religious belief will not — and should not — be accepted as part of the public morality unless they are shared by the pluarlistic community at large, by consensus."[169] The flaw here is in the *false* assumption that we are dealing with values that are derived from one particular set of religious beliefs. That makes it possible to say that the whole question of abortion can be set to one side as a religious issue. It cannot.

The Governor, like so many others, makes no reference to the clear evidence of the humanity of the embryo. I do not blame him for this. At the beginning of his talk he said that he was a lawyer and a politician and that he is not a theologian or philosopher, although he does, as one would expect, deal with both theological and philosophical concepts in his presentation. Neither is he a medical doctor nor an embryologist, but he had better deal with those issues as well. I think that he, like so many others, has been misled by the pro-abortion people who do not want us to look at embryology and so will try to insist that this is a Church-State issue, when it is not. The fact that so many religious leaders (and they are not by any stretch of the imagination all Catholic) are opposed to abortion makes it quite easy for many to discount what they say as being just "religious stuff." That is as foolish as taking Mr. Cuomo's comments as just "legal stuff" and failing to give them the hearing they deserve.

---

[168] Cuomo, *op. cit.*, pp. 6-8.

[169] Cuomo, *op. cit.*, p. 7.

Mr. Cuomo points out the fact that there are some "who say there is a simple answer to *all* these questions; they say that by history and practice of our people we were intended to be — and should be — a Christian country in law." Therefore we should impose Christian norms. He is right in rejecting any such concept. In fact, I would envision some considerable difficulty in even attempting to establish that our country could be seriously described as Christian.

The second set of answers[170] looks at the fact that what we believe to be best cannot always be put into effect and that even the modes of political persuasion vary and are not at all a matter of faith. In other words, even if new laws were the best way to proceed, and even if our faith demanded that we look toward such laws, faith would not be able to supply for everyone that best way in which he could work toward such a goal. "That is, while we always owe our Bishops' words respectful attention and careful consideration, the question whether to engage the political system in a struggle to have it adopt certain articles of our belief as part of public morality, is not a matter of doctrine: it is a matter of prudential political judgement."[171]

As he points out, "on divorce and birth control, without changing its moral teaching, the Church abides the civil law as it now stands — without making much of a point of it — that in our pluralistic society we are not required to

---

[170] Cuomo, *op. cit.*, pp. 8-13.

[171] Cuomo, *op. cit.*, p. 9.

insist that *all* our religious values be the law of the land."[172]

Do you see the same basic error in these arguments? There is the supposition that we are dealing with a matter of religious belief as opposed to civil law and the total failure to realize the truth of the matter. The reality is that we are legally killing millions of people each year because of a legalism that fails to look at the truth.

When he speaks of the Church's tolerance of civil law in regard to birth control or divorce, he is, in a sense, equating these with the issue of abortion (even though at one point he points out that abortion is a matter of life and death). His intent, as he makes clear, is not to say that all these issues are equal, but rather that just as the Church does not propose a political plan to bring about laws on divorce or birth control, so it should leave to individual politicians decisions on the best political plan to do something about abortion.

Certainly divorce is an enormous problem in our country. But the Church recognizes cases in which separation is necessary. It also recognizes cases in which there were such problems from the beginning of a marriage that the marriage was not even valid — hence the possibility of decrees of annulment. The church speaks to its own members about this, but does not presume to legislate for others.

In regard to birth control, the church does indeed teach that it is wrong, but it does not invoke the need for legal sanction for those who do it. It does talk about the need for legal restriction in regard to abortion. In the *Roe v.*

---

[172] Cuomo, *op.cit.*, p. 9.

*Wade* hearing of October, 1972, Mr. Robert C. Flowers, the attorney for the State of Texas, quoted from an earlier case in which judges had argued from the fact that the state allows birth control to the fact that it could therefore not rule against abortion. A dissenting judge wrote in the minority opinion: "In other words, in their views no distinction can be made between prohibiting the use of contraceptives and prohibiting the destruction of fetal life, which, as explained above, can be construed to be a human life. I find this assertion incredible. Contraception prevents the creation of new life; abortion destroys the existing life. Contraception and abortion are as distinguishable as thoughts and dreams are distinguishable from a reality."[173]

Abortion is a far greater evil than either divorce or birth control. It destroys innocent life. If it rarely occurred, there might be no need for a general law about it. In this Country, however, it occurs on an average of about *4000 times a day*. Someone had better do something.

Still, the Governor is right in saying that it is not the function of the Church to define a particular political plan to achieve such goals. He says: "I repeat, there is no Church teaching that mandates the best political course for making our belief everyone's rule, for spreading this part of our Catholicism. There is neither an encyclical nor a catechism that spells out a political strategy for achieving legislative goals."[174] This is his primary point in this part of the argument. It is still fatally flawed, of course, with

---

[173] Supreme court, *op. cit.*, p. 37.

[174] Cuomo, *op. cit.*, p. 11.

the notion that the abortion issue is simply a "part of our Catholicism," when in reality it is obviously more than that.

The next part of his answer[175] argues that legal interdiction of abortion by federal or state government is not a "plausible possibility" and that, even if it could be done, it wouldn't work. It would be "'Prohibition' revisited, legislating what couldn't be enforced and in the process creating a disrespect for law in general."[176] "Nor would a denial of medicaid funding for abortion achieve our objectives."[177] "The hard truth is that abortion isn't a failure of government. No agency or department of government forces women to have abortions, but abortion goes on... collectively we Catholics apparently believe — and perhaps act — little differently from those who don't share our commitment."[178] He suggests, instead, that we should and could accomplish more by the force of good example and lack of hypocrisy.[179] I could hardly argue with that. All along I have been insisting that we must not only say what is right, we must *do* it.

Beneath all the rhetoric, however, is the real crux of the whole issue. Of course the Church cannot and should not

---

[175] Cuomo, *op. cit.*, pp. 13-16.

[176] Cuomo, *op. cit.*, p. 13.

[177] *Ibid.*

[178] Cuomo, *op. cit.*, p. 14.

[179] Cf. Cuomo, *op. cit.*, p. 15.

mandate one precise political plan as though such a plan were a matter of faith. In fact, I am not aware that it has done so or ever showed signs of doing so. It has, however, attempted to make it quite clear that no one can live with two heads which disagree with each other, and still claim to be one person. It is ridiculous to say, "I am personally opposed to abortion," while saying at the same time, "I will be glad to promote abortion, or "I will be sure to do nothing to stop it." This is just the sort of hedging that many candidates try to use. It is dishonest.

When government says that abortion is a right and then even funds that right, it cannot then expect any credibility at all if it claims to be opposed to it. Some politicians would like to create the impression that they are opposed to abortion as a personal belief, but that they are law abiding citizens who *can* do nothing to stop it. Some of them really mean they *will not attempt* to do anything to stop it. There are, of course, real limits to what any *one* legislator or judge or executive may do. The very least that can be done, however, is not to promote it. The legislator who votes for pro-abortion bills or funding is doing wrong no matter what he says. He may, in good conscience and with good political reasons, vote for a bill which places further restrictions even if it does not completely prohibit abortion, since that may be the best that can be accomplished at a given time. An executive may sign such legislation into law for the same reason. The executive is in a particularly crucial position if he has the power to veto. He *can* veto bills that offer funding for abortions and he *should* do so. Of course, they may go back to the legislature and be passed over the veto. That is part of the democratic process also. The executive cannot change that; but if he fails to use his own power properly, then he should be honest enough to admit that he does indeed favor abortion and its funding.

270

Otherwise he acts to preserve his job, but he can no longer claim to be really opposed to the killing of the unborn.

The Governor argues that, in spite of *Roe v. Wade*, there is much that we can do. He says: "While we argue over abortion, the United States' infant mortality rate places us sixteenth among the nations of the world. Thousands of infants die each year because of inadequate medical care. Some are born with birth defects that, with proper treatment, could be prevented. Some are stunted in their physical and mental growth because of improper nutrition... there is work enough for all of us. Lifetimes of it."[180] What he says is true, but it is worse than foolish to imply that we can therefore ignore the question of abortion and feel good that we are doing other works. I find that as unrealistic as it was for German politicians to fund Hitler's atrocities while pointing to the prosperity that his government had brought about. There are thousands of infants who die needlessly each year. And there are 1,600,000 who are purposely murdered.

Governor Cuomo goes on to say: "Abortion has a unique significance but not a preemptive significance... Approval or rejection of legal restrictions on abortion should not be the exclusive litmus test of Catholic loyalty."[181] He is right. It should not be the *only* test, but is *one real* test. I cannot claim to be living a good life on the ground that I keep all of the commandments except one. *The commandments are not multiple choice.*

---

[180] Cuomo, *op. cit.*, p. 16.

[181] Cuomo, *op. cit.*, pp. 16-17.

What should the Bishops do in regard to Catholic politicians who clearly act in favor of abortion on demand while claiming that they are personally opposed to it? How should they react to those who make an issue of their Catholicism to get elected while, at the same time, making it clear that no one need fear them when it comes to restricting abortion? They should, it seems to me, care enough about those politicians to point out to them just how wrong they are. If they cannot or will not change, then the Bishop should not stand by in silence, thus allowing even more to be misled. He should state clearly and publicly that this person is *not* living out the truth and is *not* living out the teaching of his own Church. This is not a retreat into fundamentalism and it is not a position which will settle for nothing other than full civil implementation of its views.[182] It is the care of a pastor for his flock. "If I say to the wicked, 'you shall surely die,' and you fail to warn him — if you say nothing to warn the wicked man from his wicked way, in order to save his life — he being wicked shall die for his iniquity, but his blood will I require at your hand. If, however, you warn the wicked man, and he turn not away from his wicked conduct and his wicked way, he shall die for his iniquity, but you will have saved yourself."[183] The matter of abortion is *not* a specifically Catholic issue; but it is a matter so important and so basic

---

[182] Cf. Cuomo, *op.cit.*, p. 12.

[183] Ezekiel 3, 18-19.

272

that the Church would be remiss if it did not teach the truth and teach it with authority.[184]

As I said, it has now been six years since the Governor gave his speech. In those years there have been some changes — some for the good and some for the worse. One of these was the decision of the Supreme Court in the case of *Webster v. Reproductive Health Services.* This decision upheld a Missouri law forbidding public employees to perform or assist in abortions. It also forbade the use of public facilities in the performance of abortions and required doctors to determine, in pregnancies of 20 weeks or more, whether the baby is viable. The decision did not undo *Roe v. Wade*, but it did narrow its applications and allowed for the State to set some possible limits on the wholesale slaughter of the unborn. The limits were all too small, but they were limits.

Governor Cuomo emphasizes the oath of public officials to preserve the Constitution.[185] He is clear in his concept that an official, in his function of preserving the Constitution, should not deny funding for women to have abortions. The reason for this is, of course, *Roe v. Wade*, which is a decision of the Supreme Court and, therefore, an authentic interpretation of the Constitution. "Given *Roe v. Wade* it would be nothing more than an attempt to do indirectly

---

[184] The *Declaration on Procured Abortion* of the Congregation for the Doctrine of the Faith in 1974 had already given answers to many of Governor Cuomo's questions. The relevant passages, as translated in *Vatican Council II: More Postconciliar Documents*, Austin Flannery, *ed.*, are given in appendix II.

[185] Cf. Cuomo, *op. cit.*, p. 4.

what the law says cannot be done directly..."[186]   At the same time he says that he considers abortion wrong and is personally opposed to it.[187]  In view of all this, you might expect that the *Webster v. Reproductive Health Services* decision would give him some relief. It at least presents a way in which *some* limits can be imposed directly and with the support of the Supreme Court — that authentic interpreter of the Constitution.

The *Webster* decision was handed down on July 3, 1989. Three days later Governor Cuomo announced his intention to *reject* any legislation that would limit abortion in the ways set out by the Supreme Court![188]   Now, of course, Governor Cuomo could not make laws all by himself.  In other words, what he is saying is this: *Even if a majority of the legislators in New York presented him with a law drawn up totally in accord with the decisions of the Supreme Court, he would veto it*!  In the same speech, however, he also spoke of another Supreme Court decision which had held that "no law could prohibit political protestors from burning the American flag."[189]   He affirmed that he would find a way to ban flag-burning. There seems to me to be a seriously distorted sense of priorities

---

[186] Cuomo, *op. cit.*, p. 13.


[187] Cf. Cuomo, *op. cit.*, pp. 9-10.


[188] Cf. *The New York Times*, July 6, 1989, p. 1 and p. A 16 (reported by Elizabeth Kolbert.


[189] *Ibid.*

274

at work here. He will do his all to save the flag, while drawing no limit on abortion in a state which in 1985 (the most recent year for which statistics are available) allowed the legal murder of 195,100 babies. I have a hard time reconciling his actions with the good example of respect for unborn life of which he spoke so glowingly in 1984. It is equally hard to avoid the conclusion that he is looking not to the issues but to reelection.

We all have a right to expect our elected officials to act in accord with conscience. We have a right to expect them not to have two consciences, one public and one private. That road leads to ruin and chaos. If a person's conscience tells him that abortion is wrong, then he should say so in words and actions, public and private. If it says that abortion is acceptable, then he should say so in words and actions, public and private. He should not hide behind one or the other in order to garner votes. I cannot accuse Governor Cuomo or any other politician of doing this consciously or wilfully. I cannot see into their minds or hearts. but he and others — wittingly or unwittingly — are doing just that, and they are dead wrong. I surely would not vote for them to represent me. I would never be able to be sure just how much evil their public conscience could tolerate, and so I could never trust them. When I hear them proclaim the value of the gift of life and then watch them do nothing to preserve that gift for the most helpless members of society, I am appalled. They do not shower favors alike on the high and the low, the rich and the poor. They offer us, instead, a bitter pill to swallow, and no amount of fudge will sweeten it.

# CHAPTER 33

# THE JUSTICE IS BLIND

Atop the Old Bailey, the criminal court in London, there is (or so I have been told, not having been there to check for myself) a large statue of Justice. In one hand it holds a balance — indicating that all evidence is weighed. In the other it holds a sword — the threat of legitimate power to enforce its rule. Around its eyes is a blindfold — showing that it judges by the weight of the evidence, and not by its vision of the person who comes for judgement. It is a symbol of the fairness of law and the courts. The court Justice who hears the case, however, should keep both eyes and ears open to the evidence. If he judges on the basis of his own preconceptions — or even misconceptions — then he does not do justice. If he does not, cannot, or simply will not grasp the meaning of the issues and the evidence, then he will be blind to the truth and will fail in his mission.

This sort of blindness can affect any court, even the Supreme Court of the United States. There are good examples of it in *Webster v. Human Reproductive Services.*[190] It is present in the dissenting opinion offered by

---

[190] The texts of all of the various Justices in *Webster v. Reproductive Health Services* will be quoted from *Origins, CNS Documentary Service*, July 13, 1989, Vol. 19, No. 9, pp. 129-151. I will cite references by giving the name of the Justice who wrote the opinion and the page on which it occurs (e.g., Scalia,

Justice Harry Blackmun (and concurred in by Justices William Brennan and Thurgood Marshall). It is exemplified quite fully in the opinion written by Justice John Paul Stevens. When it comes to the question of abortion, the Justice is blind.

What is it to which these Justices are blind? It is the essential question of the humanity of the embryo. They argue the interpretation of the law without reference to whether the law reflects the truth of the matter. As I mentioned in the preceding chapter, the notion of person and the interest of the State in protection of the unborn, were framed in purely legal grounds of interpretation of amendments 5, 9 and 14 of the Constitution. Thus, the decision made in *Roe v. Wade.* However, is that not what the Supreme Court is expected to do?

In one sense, yes, it is. It is a last court of appeal for those cases, in which the laws of the various States seem to place upon citizens burdens which violate the freedom or rights which pertain to every citizen in every state by reason of constitutional guarantee.

In another sense, however, the function of the Supreme Court will always involve more than that. The Constitution is two centuries old and it is an amazingly brief document. It will always be in need of interpretation.[191] Some interpretation will involve the precise intent of articles or amendments. Some will involve the effort to discern the

---

140).

[191] The Constitution of the United States is a most astounding document. In broad, sweeping lines it established a country which has survived for more than 200 years. It has been modified by only 26 amendments, all of them relatively brief.

intent of the founding fathers. Some will involve the effort to correlate the intent of the document with new situations and new knowledge. There are also times, of course, when interpretation may not be possible because some area of concern is simply missing from the document. It may not even have been envisioned 200 years ago. In that case, the only solution left open for peaceful resolution is amendment.

In any instance of interpretation, it would be foolish to think that it will occur with cold, passionless objectivity. That is seldom the case with law, since legal conflict frequently springs from passion and is designed to subdue or overcome it, so as to maintain a peaceful society. The judges who interpret are themselves human and subject to the same passions. Every effort is made to get men who are upright and honest to serve on the Court; and I would say that, in the years of our history, we have done rather well. In areas which involve interpretation by reason of new knowledge or new insight, the Justices must also learn — and some, of course, will do better than others. That new knowledge may very well involve areas other than the law itself, and so may not be within the expertise of the lawyers who have been appointed to the Court. They may not know the answers and may not even know which questions to ask. They may, at times, get in beyond their depth. Every one of them will also come to every case with a set of personal presuppositions that will color all of the judgements that are made. We hope for the best and we frequently get it, but we also at times run into dreadful error and hope that time and future justice or amendments can correct it.

Probably one of the most dreadful errors of the last century was in the Dred Scott case. It was on March 6 of 1857 that the Court decided that congress could not bar

278

slavery from a territory, that a slave still remained a slave even if taken into a free state and that blacks could not be citizens. The vote was 7-2. I have no doubt that the seven Justices (including Chief Justice Roger B. Taney) were convinced that they were right and were probably sure that they had been completely objective. We can look back now and see their action as wrong and unjust. It was, without doubt, influenced by political expediency, ignorance, bias against blacks, lack of necessary knowledge and insight, and a dreadful flaw in the Constitution itself. It took an amendment to undo it, and it took a bloody civil war to bring about that amendment. It was a decision not to help the helpless and, as such, was immoral. But it was legal, legally binding and a perfect example of the worst kind of legalism. We should not, however, be so naive as to think that it was a fluke and could never happen again. The human failings which afflicted that court can just as easily afflict any and every court.

Does *Roe v. Wade* really parallel the travesty of justice that was perpetrated in *Dred Scott*? Justice Blackmun clearly tries to avoid the parallel. I would suspect that he would be aware of the fact that the comparison has so frequently been made. He is, I have no doubt, aware of the fact that *Dred Scott* needed to be reversed and was indeed reversed, not only by amendment, but by implication in almost every subsequent Supreme Court decision in the area of civil rights. He sees the decision in *Webster v. Reproductive Health Services* as the beginning of an overturning of *Roe v. Wade.* He says:

> Of the aspirations and settled understanding of
> American women, of the inevitable and brutal
> consequences of what it is doing, the tough-ap-
> proach plurality utters not a word. This silence is

callous. It is also profoundly destructive of this court as an institution. To overturn a constitutional decision is a rare and grave undertaking. To overturn a constitutional decision that secured a fundamental personal liberty to millions of persons would be unprecedented in our 200 years of constitutional history.[192]

First of all, a decision that is blatantly wrong deserves to be overturned and at the earliest opportunity. Such is *Roe v. Wade*, which has opened up the way to considering a whole category of millions of persons as disposable tissue, available for death, experiment and to serve as the raw material for lucrative businesses. The Justice, of course, looks at it from another perspective. He sees *Roe v. Wade* as a guarantee of fundamental rights for women. He ignores the unborn and rejects them as persons. His eyes are open only to what he sees as a violation of women's rights. Thus, in his view, to overturn *Roe v. Wade* is unthinkable.

What might he say of *Dred Scott*? It would not surprise me even a little to learn that he considered it a dreadful decision, deserving to be overturned. It was not a decision for freedom, but against it. But would its formulators have allowed him or anyone else to get away with that? I should think not. They would, no doubt, have said that *Dred Scott* should never be overturned. It had secured for slave owners the fundamental personal liberty to their own free ownership of property. The government had no right to intervene. Slave owners and slave traders could all agree on that, and they could drum up a lot of support among

---

[192] Blackmun, 145.

others by saying that any reversal would be a dire threat to the future freedom of everyone. All of this made sense, provided that slaves were never viewed as persons. Once they were, of course, the whole rationale of *Dred Scott* is seen for what it is — blindness to facts combined with the worst aspects of legalism. The decision was a national shame and deserved to be consigned to oblivion.

The same can be said for *Roe v. Wade.* It guarantees the "rights" of one group at the expense of rejection, not only of the rights, but even of the lives of others. It, too, deserves to be consigned to oblivion.

The Missouri law had contained provision that required the physician not to abort a viable fetus. It also said that when the fetal age has reached 20 weeks, the physician would be required to perform the tests that would indicate whether the unborn child was viable or not. Viability, of course, occurs at 23 1/2 or 24 weeks of age. It is not, however, at all uncommon for estimates of fetal age to be off by as much as four weeks. Justice Blackmun was unhappy with this. He wrote:

By mandating tests to determine fetal weight and lung maturity for every fetus thought to be more than 20 weeks gestational age, the statute required physicians to undertake procedures, such as amniocentesis, that, in the situation presented have no medical justification, impose significant additional health risks on both the pregnant woman and the fetus, and bear no rational relation to the state's interest in protecting fetal life. As written, Section 188.029 is an arbitrary imposition of discomfort, risk and expense, furthering no discernible interest

281

except to make the procurement of an abortion as arduous and difficult as possible.[193]

It is the same Justice Blackmun, in this same document, who also writes: "No one contests that under the *Roe* framework the state, in order to promote its interest in potential human life, may regulate and even proscribe non-therapeutic abortions once the fetus becomes viable."[194] Missouri, in this law, is attempting to exercise its right to protect the viable unborn. (It should protect them even before that, but *Roe v. Wade* prevents it.) It recognizes that the viable child in question is in the womb of a woman who would like to kill it, and she and the child are being examined by a doctor who makes a living by killing fetuses. There is no doubt that it should demand proof of non-viability or viability. The word of the participants is, to say the least, rather suspect. It is also a fact that the tests mentioned in the law are not extraordinary at all. They are the same ones that would be used by a doctor to determine viability if he were trying to save a child who had to be delivered prematurely.

As to Justice Blackmun's fears that the tests would be dangerous to mother and fetus, they are ridiculous. The risks to the mother at this stage of pregnancy would be minimal (apart from sloppy doctors). At this stage, too, the risks to the fetus are far less than in earlier weeks. The Justice, however, seems to have left all logic somewhere behind him when he expresses concern that the fetus runs a risk in the test, when he knows full well that without the

---

[193] Blackmun, 142.

[194] Blackmun, 142.

282

test it will be killed.  The biggest dangers to the fetus at this point are its mother and her abortionist.

These are but a few of the flaws in the stand taken by Justice Blackmun.  There are some others as well, some of which he shares with Justice John Paul Stevens.  At this point, therefore, I will turn to what he has to say.

Justice Stevens' problems with the Missouri law begin with the fact that the preamble to the law contains "findings" of the state legislature which state that the "life of each human being begins at conception."  Upon this it bases its statement that "unborn children have protectable interests in life, health and well-being."  The Justice is even more displeased to find that the statute "commands that state laws shall be construed to provide the maximum protection to 'the unborn child at every stage of development.'"[195]  He is upset to think that the law is intended to protect the potential life of the fetus, rather than to safeguard maternal health.  Of course, he does not accept the fact that the fetus is a human person, and so he sees it as without real rights.  In that case its needs mean nothing.  The mother can abort without any reason at all, apart from the fact that she just desires to do so.  It would not occur to him that a law could try to care for both mother and child.  He also makes no point of the fact that protection of the fetus, in most instances, will not be in any way in conflict with safeguarding the health of the mother.  It may thwart her desire, but it won't hurt her health.

He is annoyed that the Missouri statute "defines *conception* as 'the fertilization of the ovum of a female by the sperm of a male... even [says Justice Stevens] standard

---

[195] Stevens, 148.

medical texts equate *conception* with implantation in the uterus occurring about six days after fertilization."[196] There are, of course, those who equate implantation with the start of pregnancy, but, to the best of my knowledge I have not come across any doctors I have ever met who would think that conception and implantation were the same thing. However, I thought, I'm willing to learn. Let's look it up. I had the *Merk Manual* handy and, when I turned to page 1743 (in the 1987 [15TH] edition), I found no confusion at all. Conception was defined as the moment of fertilization — and was quite distinct from implantation. However, the Justice uses his misinformation in a rather serious way.

If he can define conception as implantation, then he can also define contraception to mean *not* "prevention of fertilization," but "prevention of implantation." He prefers this, of course, as do so many others, because then IUD's and "morning-after pills" can be called contraceptive rather than abortifacient (and indeed they are abortifacient, as you can easily discover for yourself by looking up relevant sections in the *Physicians' Desk Reference*).

In 1965 the decision in *Griswold v. Connecticut*, on the basis of the Fourteenth Amendment's guarantee of liberty under the doctrine of due process, a Connecticut law forbidding the sale of contraceptives was overturned. Justice Stevens argues that the Missouri law is unconstitutional because its preamble would then consider IUD's and morning-after pills as abortives rather than contraceptives. It is a ridiculous piece of circular argumentation which he attempts to escape by trying to redefine conception.

---

[196] Stevens, 148.

Of course, he realizes the error in this and makes a valiant effort to head it off at the pass. He writes:

One might argue that the *Griswold* holding applies to devices "preventing conception," 381 U.S., at 480 — that is, fertilization — but not to those preventing implantation, and therefore that *Griswold* does not protect a woman's choice to use an IUD or take a morning-after pill. There is unquestionably a theological basis for such an argument, just as there was unquestionably a theological basis for the Connecticut statute that the Court invalidated in *Griswold.* Our jurisdiction, however, has consistently required a secular basis for valid legislation. Because I am not aware of any secular basis for differentiating between contraceptive procedures that are effective immediately before and those that are effective after fertilization, I believe it inescapably follows that the preamble to the Missouri statute is invalid under *Griswold* and its progeny.[197]

First of all, he says that there is an unquestionable *theological* basis for the distinction between preventing fertilization and preventing implantation. He annotates this remark, but when you read the note, what you find is this: "Several *amici* state that 'the sanctity of human life from conception and opposition to abortion are, in fact, sincere and deeply held religious beliefs.'"[198] On that sort of basis, you could equally well argue that laws against murder, rape and theft should all be overthrown because they represent sincere and deeply held religious beliefs.

---

[197] Stevens, 148.

[198] Stevens, 150, endnote 9.

He does, of course, go on to say that he is not aware of any secular basis for distinguishing between contraceptive procedures that are effective immediately before fertilization and those that are effective immediately after. Obviously part of his problem comes from the fact that he has redefined conception. The proper definition — secular or theological — is identical to the definition of fertilization. Procedures which prevent fertilization are, therefore, contraceptive. Those which prevent the fertilized ovum from implanting are not contraceptive, since they do not prevent conception. Justice Stevens would prefer that it were different, but it is not.

He does try to get out of the various inaccuracies by adding another paragraph to show what he considers the real basis for his rejection of the preamble. He says:

> Indeed I am persuaded that the absences of any secular purpose for the legislative declaration that life begins at conception and that conception occurs at fertilization makes the relevant portion of the preamble invalid under the establishment clause of the First Amendment to the Federal Constitution. This conclusion does not, and could not, rest on the fact that the statement happens to coincide with the tenets of certain religions,... or on the fact that the legislators who voted to enact it may have been motivated by religious considerations... Rather, it rests on the fact that the preamble, an unequivocal endorsement of a religious tenet of some but by no means all Christian faiths, serves no identifiable secular purpose. That fact alone compels a conclu-

sion that the statute violates the establishment clause.[199]

He recognizes here the fact that the content of the preamble *happens* to coincide with tenets of certain religions, but that this cannot invalidate it — although he seemed to be implying just the opposite of that in the passages I quoted earlier. Instead, he says that he can recognize "no secular purpose" in the content of the preamble. I'm surprised he can't. I can, and so can anyone else who thinks about it. First of all, the statement that human life begins at conception (i.e., at the moment of fertilization) is *not* a mere religious tenet. This is a simple fact based on scientific evidence, as I have already made clear. That such a human being is a *person* is a direct inference from that evidence. The *Roe v. Wade* decision ignored that and based its conclusions on a narrow minded legalism that denied basic rights to a broad category of persons under the guise of granting rights to another group. One clear secular purpose of the preamble could be to attempt to recognize that the State has an obligation to the welfare of all its members, even the unborn. And this is so even if the decision of a court unjustly deprives the several states of their capacity to protect those rights. There is, in fact, a most urgent secular need for recognition of the truth.

Again in his annotation Justice Stevens makes a most interesting remark. He says:

Pointing to the lack of consensus about life's onset among experts in medicine, philosophy and theology, the court in *Roe v. Wade*,... established that the Constitution does not permit a state to adopt a theory of life

---

[199] Stevens, 148-149.

that overrides a pregnant woman's rights... The constitutional violation is doubly grave if, as here, the only basis for the state's "finding" is non-secular.[200]

This sounds as though it makes some sense, until you realize that the Court, in its decision, was perfectly willing to choose among theories. It chose the one that ignored all the evidence and denied rights to the unborn child. It compounded its folly by trying to use its trimester notion to recover some of its credibility. It did not succeed.

Justice Stevens turns to the writings of St. Thomas Aquinas to make his point. Although I have addressed this in an earlier chapter,[201] I would like to add some comments here also. Thomas' idea that the male soul develops at 40 days and the female soul at 80, was *not* in itself a theological doctrine. It was the *scientific* knowledge of the Thirteenth Century, based on very limited means of observation. It represented the earliest stages at which science and medicine could observe the human appearance and the sexual differentiation of the fetus. The concept of the fetus as "seed" and as "formed" was also based on scientific concepts. The male seed was planted in the uterus and grew, eventually taking on human form and so becoming human life — described in terms of having a soul. When the Church legislated about abortion, therefore, its penalties were clearly going to be more severe after the fetus was "formed" than they were before.

As time went on, science became increasingly more sophisticated in its methods of observation, even down to

---

[200] Stevens, 150, endnote 12.

[201] Cf. *supra*, chapter 9.

the genetic structure of the earliest stages of the embryo. Science grew in its grasp of the continuity of human life. Medicine grew in its knowledge of embryology and fetology, learning that many characteristics of the newborn, or even of the adult, can be traced back to the fertilized ovum — the first moment of a continuous life. From all of this the Church also learned and realized that its view on the start of personal life was too limited. It learned that abortion at any stage from conception onward was murder. In fact, it seems that everyone learned — except some members of the Supreme Court.

Justice Stevens says that, if St. Thomas' views were held, we might get a "finding" that female life begins at 80 days and male life at 40. The court, he says, would promptly conclude that a law with such a "particular religious tenet" would surely be rejected by the Court as a violation of the establishment clause of the First Amendment.[202]   He concludes:

> In my opinion the difference between that hypothetical statute and Missouri's preamble reflects nothing more than a difference in theological doctrine.[203]

*He is utterly wrong.* What he is dealing with is *not* a theological doctrine. There is a vast difference in *scientific evidence and scientific conclusions.* Actually, there is very little difference in the theology, which says, from the time of St. Thomas Aquinas until now, that it is wrong to murder human beings — a position which any state or any of its courts ought to adopt as well.

---

[202] Cf. Stevens, 149.

[203] Stevens, 149.

Justice Stevens also says that there is an obvious difference between the state interest in the fertilized ovum and the nine-month fetus on the eve of birth.

"There can be no interest in protecting the newly fertilized egg from physical pain or mental anguish, because the capacity for such suffering does not yet exist; respecting a developed fetus, however, that interest is valid."[204] On this ground, of course, the state should have no interest either in the unconscious or comatose patient, who also has no capacity for physical pain or mental anguish. That would be a stupid conclusion so Justice Stevens' principle, from which it is clearly derived, must be a stupid principle.

At the end of his argument, Justice Stevens says, "To paraphrase St. Thomas — until a seed has acquired the powers of sensation and movement, the life of a human being has not yet begun."[205] I, for one, am not satisfied to base my conclusion on Thirteenth Century science. Apparently Justice Stevens is. The Justice is blind.

---

[204] Stevens, 149.

[205] Stevens, 150.

290

## DEATH OR LIFE??

The Iraqis bother us. "Nuke 'em." My baby has Down's Syndrome. "Abort it." My mother is in a coma. "Pull the plug." I cannot afford another child. "Kill it." There are criminals everywhere. "Execute them." My child cries too much. "Beat it to death." I have a prowler. "Shoot him." I have Alzheimer's. "Kill yourself." I can't stand the pain. "Commit suicide."

Is death the answer to everything in our society? It may sometimes seem that way. Perhaps we watch too much television, where every problem is solved in 30 to 60 minutes, the dead bodies are carted away in sanitary fashion during the commercials, those who are beaten or injured are back in full health by the next episode without so much as a scratch and the good guys always win. Action takes the place of dialogue, visual imagery takes the place of writing, shallow sex takes the place of any depth of love. It is a world of fantasy in which violence is exciting, promiscuity is fun and no one really gets hurt, people bounce in and out of marriages as though they all lived on trampolines, and the happiest marriages are those not bothered by children.

It is an unreal world in which we exist as passive observers, feeling only vicarious pain (which doesn't really hurt at all beyond the occasional teardrop) and vicarious pleasure (which lasts only until the station break). World events — even the most atrocious — are brought in living color right into our living rooms. You can enjoy your supper while watching views of airline crashes, victims of bombing, gory accidents and hostages hanged for publicity value. You can be so desensitized that what would once have made you ill now becomes background noise during your evening hour to unwind from the rigors of the day. World issues are summarized in one minute spots — film at eleven — and the most complex problems must be reduced to slogans. You need not think. All ideas have been predigested and are given to you in small, bite-size morsels. You can be pro-choice (which will allow you the freedom to kill someone now and again) or you can be pro-life (which will allow you never to see a fair presentation of the facts in most of the media). To every problem that faces you, you can draw your weapon and say, "Go ahead. Make my day."

Real life is much harder, but it is also infinitely better. Its rewards are real and are guaranteed by God Himself not to fade away. Respect for life makes demands in many ways, but it also makes for something more than temporary self-satisfaction. The living of life has purpose and it becomes far too precious to waste.

In this book I have tried to focus on life and love. The basis for what I have said is, to a large extent, given in the *Instruction on Procreation*. There, in the rather formal and sometimes technical language of such documents, is a vision that can open our eyes to the reality of life itself. All I have tried to do in this book is to translate some of that vision into words that may be easier to understand. To make the vision a reality, we must also open our minds to the truth and our hearts to the good. We cannot remain passive observers. We must know, speak and act the true.

292

"With this Instruction the Congregation for the Doctrine of the Faith, in fulfilling its responsibility to promote and defend the Church's teaching in so serious a matter, addresses a new and heartfelt invitation to all those who, by reason of their role and their commitment, can exercise a positive influence and ensure that, in the family and in society, due respect is accorded to life and love. It addresses this invitation to those responsible for the formation of consciences and of public opinion, to scientists and medical professionals, to jurists and politicians. It hopes that all will understand the incompatibility between recognition of the dignity of the human person and contempt for life and love, between faith in the living God and the claim to decide arbitrarily the origin and fate of a human being."

We are *all* called to life and love. God's most precious gifts have been put into our hands. This does not make us their owners; we are, rather, their stewards. We have a responsibility to care for what we are given and to place it back into the hands of the real Owner when this life is done. In the meantime, they are not given simply so that we can keep them for ourselves, but so that we can communicate them to others. In order for that actually to happen, we must believe and we must understand. We must learn and we must communicate. We must make decisions, often hard ones, and we must live out what we know to be true. In our present world this will be, at times, a trial. In much of what we do and say, we will be facing and making choices which touch on matters of life and death. Choose life.

# APPENDIX I

Congregation for the Doctrine of the Faith
INSTRUCTION
ON
**RESPECT FOR HUMAN LIFE IN ITS ORIGIN
AND ON THE DIGNITY OF PROCREATION**
REPLIES TO CERTAIN QUESTIONS OF THE DAY

## FOREWORD

*The Congregation for the Doctrine of the Faith has
been approached by various Episcopal Conferences or
individual Bishops, by theologians, doctors and scientists, concerning biomedical techniques which make it
possible to intervene in the initial phase of the life of a
human being and in the very processes of procreation
and their conformity with the principles of Catholic
morality. The present Instruction, which is the result of
wide consultation and in particular of a careful evaluation of the declarations made by Episcopates, does not
intend to repeat all the Church's teaching on the dignity
of human life as it originates and on procreation, but to
offer, in the light of the previous teaching of the Magisterium, some specific replies to the main questions being
asked in this regard.*

*The exposition is arranged as follows: an introduction
will recall the fundamental principles, of an anthropological and moral character, which are necessary for a
proper evaluation of the problems and for working out
replies to those questions; the first part will have as its
subject respect for the human being from the first
moment of his or her existence; the second part will
deal with the moral questions raised by technical
interventions on human procreation; the third part will*

*offer some orientations on the relationships between moral law and civil law in terms of the respect due to human embryos and foetuses* and as regard the legitimacy of techniques of artificial procreation.*

## INTRODUCTION
## 1.
## BIOMEDICAL RESEARCH AND THE TEACHING OF THE CHURCH

1. The gift of life which God the Creator and Father has entrusted to man calls him to appreciate the inestimable value of what he has been given and to take responsibility for it: this fundamental principle must be placed at the center of one's reflection in order to clarify and solve the moral problems raised by artificial interventions on life as it originates and on the processes of procreation.

2. Thanks to the progress of the biological and medical sciences, man has at his disposal ever more effective therapeutic resources; but he can also acquire new powers, with unforeseeable consequences, over human life at its very beginning and in its first stages. Various procedures now make it possible to intervene not only in order to assist but also to dominate the processes of procreation. These techniques can enable man to "take in hand his own

---

*The terms "zygote," "pre-embryo," "embryo" and "foetus" can indicate in the vocabulary of biology successive stages of the development of a human being. The present Instruction makes free use of these terms, attributing to them an identical ethical relevance, in order to designate the result (whether visible or not) of human generation, from the first moment of its existence until birth. The reason for this usage is clarified by the text (cf I, 1).

destiny," but they also expose him "to the temptation to go beyond the limits of a reasonable dominion over nature."[1] They might constitute progress in the service of man, but they also involve serious risks. Many people are therefore expressing an urgent appeal that in interventions on procreation the values and rights of the human person be safeguarded. Requests for clarification and guidance are coming not only from the faithful but also from those who recognize the Church as "an expert in humanity"[2] with a mission to serve the "civilization of love"[3] and of life.

3. The Church's Magisterium does not intervene on the basis of a particular competence in the area of the experimental sciences; but having taken account of the data of research and technology, it intends to put forward, by virtue of its evangelical mission and apostolic duty, the moral teaching corresponding to the dignity of the person and to his or her integral vocation. It intends to do so by expounding the criteria of moral judgment as regards the applications of scientific research and technology, especially in relation to human life and its beginnings. These criteria are the respect, defense and promotion of man, his "primary

---

[1] POPE JOHN PAUL II. *Discourse to those taking part in the 81st Congress of the Italian Society of Internal Medicine and the 82nd Congress of the Italian Society of General Surgery*, 27 October 1980: AAS 72 (1980) 1126.

[2] POPE PAUL VI, *Discourse to the general Assembly of the United Nations Organization*, 4 October 1965: AAS 57 (1965) 878; Encyclical *Populorum Progressio*, 13: AAS 59 (1967) 263.

[3] POPE PAUL VI, *Homily during the Mass closing the Holy Year*, 25 December 1975: AAS 68 (1976) 145; POPE JOHN PAUL II, Encyclical *Dives in Misericordia*, 30: AAS 72 (1980) 1224.

and fundamental right" to life,[4] his dignity as a person who is endowed with a spiritual soul and with moral responsibility[5] and who is called to beatific communion with God.

4. The Church's intervention in this field is inspired also by the love which she owes to man, helping him to recognize and respect his rights and duties. This love draws from the fount of Christ's love: as she contemplates the mystery of the Incarnate Word, the Church also comes to understand the "mystery of man";[6] by proclaiming the Gospel of salvation, she reveals to man his dignity and invites him to discover fully the truth of his own being. Thus the Church once more puts forward the divine law in order to accomplish the work of truth and liberation.

5. For it is out of goodness — in order to indicate the path of life — that God gives human beings his commandments and the grace to observe them: and it is likewise out of goodness — in order to help them persevere along the same path — that God always offers to everyone his forgiveness. Christ has compassion on our weaknesses: he is our Creator and Redeemer. May his spirit open men's hearts to the gift of God's peace and to an understanding of his precepts.

---

[4] POPE JOHN PAUL II, *Discourse to those taking part in the 35th General Assembly of the World Medical Association*, 29 October 1983: AAS 76 (1984) 390.

[5] CF Declaration *Dignitatis Humanae*, 2.

[6] Pastoral Constitution *Gaudium et Spes*, 22; POPE JOHN PAUL II, Encyclical *Redemptor Hominis*, 8: AAS 71 (1979) 270-272.

# 2.
## SCIENCE AND TECHNOLOGY
## AT THE SERVICE OF THE HUMAN PERSON

6.  God created man in his own image and likeness: "male and female he created them" (Gen 1:27), entrusting to them the task of "having dominion over the earth" (Gen 1:28). Basic scientific research and applied research constitute a significant expression of this dominion of man over creation. Science and technology are valuable resources for man when placed at his service and when they promote his integral development for the benefit of all; but they cannot of themselves show the meaning of existence and of human progress. Being ordered to man, who initiates and develops them, they draw from the person and his moral values the indication of their purpose and the awareness of their limits.

7.  It would on the one hand be illusory to claim that scientific research and its applications are morally neutral; on the other hand one cannot derive criteria for guidance from mere technical efficiency, from research's possible usefulness to some at the expense of others, or, worse still, from prevailing ideologies. Thus science and technology require, for their own intrinsic meaning, an unconditional respect for the fundamental criteria of the moral law: that is to say, they must be at the service of the human person, of his inalienable rights and his true and integral good according to the design and will of God.[7]

8. The rapid development of technological discoveries gives greater urgency to this need to respect the criteria just mentioned: science without conscience can only lead to

---

[7]Cf. Pastoral Constitution *Gaudium et Spes*, 35.

man's ruin. "Our era needs such wisdom more than bygone ages if the discoveries made by man are to be further humanized. For the future of the world stands in peril unless wiser people are forthcoming".[8]

### 3.
### ANTHROPOLOGY AND PROCEDURES
### IN THE BIOMEDICAL FIELD

9. Which moral criteria must be applied in order to clarify the problems posed today in the field of biomedicine? The answer to this question presupposes a proper idea of the nature of the human person in his bodily dimension.

10. For it is only in keeping with his true nature that the human person can achieve self-realization as a "unified totality":[9] and this nature is at the same time corporal and spiritual. By virtue of its substantial union with a spiritual soul, the human body cannot be considered as a mere complex of tissues, organs and functions, nor can it be evaluated in the same way as the body of animals; rather it is a constitutive part of the person who manifests and expresses himself through it.

11. The natural moral law expresses and lays down the purposes, rights and duties which are based upon the bodily and spiritual nature of the human person. Therefore this

---

[8] Pastoral Constitution *Gaudium et Spes*, 15; cf. also POPE PAUL VI, Encyclical *Populorum Progressio*, 20: AAS 59 (1967) 267; POPE JOHN PAUL II, Encyclical *Redemptor Hominis*, 15: AAS 71 (1979) 286-289); Apostolic Exhortation *Familiaris Consortio*, 8: AAS 74 (1982) 89.

[9] POPE JOHN PAUL II, Apostolic Exhortation *Familiaris Consortio*, 11: AAS 74 (1982) 92.

law cannot be thought of as simply a set of norms on the biological level; rather it must be defined as the rational order whereby man is called by the Creator to direct and regulate his life and actions and in particular to make use of his own body.[10]

12. A first consequence can be deduced from these principles: an intervention on the human body affects not only the tissues, the organs and their functions but also involves the person himself on different levels. It involves, therefore, perhaps in an implicit but nonetheless real way, a moral significance and responsibility. Pope John Paul II forcefully reaffirmed this to the World Medical Association when he said: "Each human person, in his absolutely unique singularity, is constituted not only by his spirit, but by his body as well. Thus, in the body and through the body, one touches the person himself in his concrete reality. To respect the dignity of man consequently amounts to safeguarding this identify of the man *'corpore et anima unus,'* as the Second Vatican Council says (*Gaudium et Spes,* 14 par. 1). It is on the basis of this anthropological vision that one is to find the fundamental criteria for decision making in the case of procedures which are not strictly therapeutic, as, for example, those aimed at the improvement of the human biological condition.[11]

13. Applied biology and medicine work together for the integral good of human life when they come to the aid of

---

[10] Cf. POPE PAUL VI, Encyclical *Humanae Vitae,* 10: AAS 60 (1968) 487-488.

[11] POPE JOHN PAUL II, *Discourse to the members of the 35th General Assembly of the World Medical Association,* 29 October 1983: AAS 76 (1984) 393.

a person stricken by illness and infirmity and when they respect his or her dignity as a creature of God. No biologist or doctor can reasonably claim, by virtue of his scientific competence, to be able to decide on people's origin and destiny. This norm must be applied in a particular way in the field of sexuality and procreation, in which man and woman actualize the fundamental values of love and life.

14.   God, who is love and life, has inscribed in man and woman the vocation to share in a special way in his mystery of personal communion and in his work as Creator and Father.[12]   For this reason marriage possesses specific goods and values in its union and in procreation which cannot be likened to those existing in lower forms of life. Such values and meaning are of the personal order and determine from the moral point of view the meaning and limits of artificial interventions on procreation and on the origin of human life.   These interventions are not to be rejected on the grounds that they are artificial.   As such, they bear witness to the possibilities of the art of medicine. but they must be given a moral evaluation in reference to the dignity of the human person, who is called to realize his vocation from God to the gift of love and the gift of life.

## 4.
## FUNDAMENTAL CRITERIA FOR A MORAL JUDG-MENT

15.   The fundamental values connected with the techniques

---

[12] Cf. POPE JOHN PAUL II, Apostolic Exhortation *Familiaris Consortio*, 11: AAS 74 (1982) 91-92; cf. also Pastoral Constitution *Gaudium et Spes*, 50.

of artificial human procreation are two: the life of the human being called into existence and the special nature of the transmission of human life in marriage. The moral judgment on such methods of artificial procreation must therefore be formulated in reference to these values.

16. Physical life, with which the course of human life in the world begins, certainly does not itself contain the whole of a person's value, nor does it represent the supreme good of man who is called to eternal life. However it does constitute in a certain way the "fundamental" value of life, precisely because upon this physical life all the other values of the person are based and developed.[13] The inviolability of the innocent human being's right to life "from the moment of conception until death"[14] is a sign and requirement of the very inviolability of the person to whom the Creator has given the gift of life.

17. By comparison with the transmission of other forms of life in the universe, the transmission of human life has a special character of its own, which derives from the special nature of the human person. "The transmission of human life is entrusted by nature to a personal and conscious act and as such is subject to the all-holy laws of God: immutable and inviolable laws which must be recognized and observed. For this reason one cannot use means and follow methods which could be licit in the transmission

---

[13] SACRED CONGREGATION FOR THE DOCTRINE OF THE FAITH, *Declaration on Procured Abortion, 9*, AAS 66 (1974) 736-737.

[14] POPE JOHN PAUL II, *Discourse to those taking part in the 35th General Assembly of the World Medical Association*, 29 October 1983: AAS 76 (1984) 390.

of the life of plants and animals".[15]

18.    Advances in technology have now made it possible to procreate apart from sexual relations through the meeting *in vitro* of the germ-cells previously taken from the man and the woman.  But what is technically possible is not for that very reason morally admissible.  Rational reflection on the fundamental values of life and of human procreation is therefore indispensable for formulating a moral evaluation of such technological interventions on a human being from the first stage of his development.

5.

## TEACHING OF THE MAGISTERIUM

19.    On its part, the Magisterium of the Church offers to human reason in this field too the light of Revelation: the doctrine concerning man taught by the Magisterium contains many elements which throw light on the problems being faced here.

20.    From the moment of conception, the life of every human being is to be respected in an absolute way because man is the only creature on earth that God has "wished for himself"[16] and the spiritual soul of each man is "immediately created" by God;[17] his whole being bears the image

---

[15] POPE JOHN XXIII, Encyclical *Mater et Magistra*, III:  AAS 53 (1961) 447.

[16] Pastoral Constitution *Gaudium et Spes*, 24.

[17] Cf. POPE PIUS XII, Encyclical *Humani Generis*: AAS 42 (1950) 575; POPE PAUL VI, *Professio Fidei*:  AAS 60 (1968) 436.

of the Creator. Human life is sacred because from its beginning it involves "the creative action of God"[18] and it remains forever in a special relationship with the Creator, who is its sole end.[19] God alone is the Lord of life from its beginning until its end: no one can, in any circumstance, claim for himself the right to destroy directly an innocent human being.[20]

21. Human procreation requires on the part of the spouses responsible collaboration with the fruitful love of God;[21] the gift of human life must be actualized in marriage through the specific and exclusive acts of husband and wife, in accordance with the laws inscribed in their persons and in their union.[22]

---

[18] POPE JOHN XXIII, Encyclical *Mater et Magistra*, III: AAS 53 (1961) 447; cf. POPE JOHN PAUL II, *Discourse to priests participating in a seminar on "Responsible Procreation"*, 17 September 1983, *Insegnamenti di Giovanni Paolo II*, Vi, 2 (1983) 562: "At the origin of each human person there is a creative act of God: no man comes into existence by chance; he is always the result of the creative love of God".

[19] Cf. Pastoral Constitution *Gaudium et Spes*, 24.

[20] Cf. Pope Pius XII, *Discourse to the Saint Luke Medical-Biological Union*, 12 November 1944: *Discorsi e Radiomessagi* VI (1944-1945) 191-192.

[21] Cf. Pastoral Constitution *Gaudium et Spes*, 50.

[22] Cf. Pastoral Constitution *Gaudium et Spes*, 51: "When it is a question of harmonizing married love with the responsible transmission of life, the moral character of one's behavior does not depend only on the good intention and the evaluation of the motives: the objective criteria must be used, criteria drawn from the nature of the human person and human acts, criteria which respect the total meaning of mutual self-giving and human procreation in the context of true love".

# I
## RESPECT FOR HUMAN EMBRYOS

22.  Careful reflection on this teaching of the Magisterium and on the evidence of reason, as mentioned above, enables us to respond to the numerous moral problems posed by technical interventions upon the human being in the first phases of his life and upon the process of his conception.

## 1. WHAT RESPECT IS DUE TO THE HUMAN EMBRYO, TAKING INTO ACCOUNT HIS NATURE AND IDENTITY?

*The human being must be respected — as a person — from the very first instant of his existence.*

23.  The implementation of procedures of artificial fertilization has made possible various interventions upon embryos and human foetuses.  The aims pursued are of various kinds:  diagnostic and therapeutic, scientific and commercial.  From all of this serious problems arise.  Can one speak of a right to experimentation upon human embryos for the purpose of scientific research?  What norms or laws should be worked out with regard to this matter?  The response to these problems presupposes a detailed reflection on the nature and specific identity — the word "status" is used — of the human embryo itself.
24.  At the Second Vatican Council, the Church for her part presented once again to modern man her constant and certain doctrine according to which: "Life once conceived, must be protected with the utmost care; abortion and

infanticide are abominable crimes".[23]   More recently, the
*Charter of the Rights of the Family*, published by the Holy
See, confirmed that "Human life must be absolutely
respected and protected from the moment of conception."[24]
25.   This Congregation is aware of the current debates
concerning the beginning of human life, concerning the
individuality of the human being and concerning the
identity of the human person.  The Congregation recalls the
teachings found in the *Declaration on Procured Abortion*:
"From the time that the ovum is fertilized, a new life is
begun which is neither that of the father nor of the mother;
it is rather the life of a new human being with his own
growth.   It would never be made human if it were not
human already.   To this perpetual evidence... modern
genetic science brings valuable confirmation.   It has
demonstrated that, from the first instant, the programme is
fixed as to what this living being will be:  a man, this
individual-man with his characteristic aspects already well
determined.  Right from fertilization is begun the adventure
of a human life, and each of its great capacities requires
time... to find its place and to be in a position to act".[25]
This teaching remains valid and is further confirmed, if
confirmation were needed, by recent findings of human

[23] Pastoral Constitution *Gaudium et Spes*, 51.

[24] HOLY SEE, *Charter of the Rights of the Family*, 4: *L'Osservatore Romano*,
25 November 1983.

[25] SACRED CONGREGATION FOR THE DOCTRINE OF THE FAITH,
*Declaration on Procured Abortion*, 12-13:  AAS 66 (1974) 738.

biological science which recognize that in the zygote resulting from fertilization the biological identity of a new human individual is already constituted.

26. Certainly no experimental datum can be in itself sufficient to bring us to the recognition of a spiritual soul; nevertheless, the conclusions of science regarding the human embryo provide a valuable indication for discerning by the use of reason a personal presence at the moment of this first appearance of a human life: how could a human individual not be a human person? The Magisterium has not expressly committed itself to an affirmation of a philosophical nature, but it constantly reaffirms the moral condemnation of any kind of procured abortion. This teaching has not been changed and is unchangeable.[26]

27. Thus the fruit of human generation, from the first moment of its existence, that is to say from the moment the zygote has formed, demands the unconditional respect that is morally due to the human being in his bodily and spiritual totality. The human being is to be respected and treated as a person from the moment of conception; and therefore from that same moment his rights as a person must be recognized, among which in the first place is the inviolable right of every innocent human being to life.

28. This doctrinal reminder provides the fundamental criterion for the solution of the various problems posed by the development of the biomedical sciences in this field: since the embryo must be treated as a person, it must also

---

*The Zygote is the cell produced when the nuclei of the two gametes have fused.

[26] Cf. POPE PAUL VI, *Discourse to participants in the Twenty-third National Congress of Italian Catholic Jurists*, 9 December 1972: AAS 64 (1972) 777.

be defended in its integrity, tended and cared for, to the extent possible, in the same way as any other human being as far as medical assistance is concerned.

## 2. IS PRENATAL DIAGNOSIS MORALLY LICIT?

29. *If prenatal diagnosis respects the life and integrity of the embryo and the human foetus and is directed towards its safeguarding or healing as an individual, then the answer is affirmative.*

30. For prenatal diagnosis makes it possible to know the condition of the embryo and of the foetus when still in the mother's womb. It permits, or makes it possible to anticipate earlier and more effectively, certain therapeutic, medical or surgical procedures.

31. Such diagnosis is permissible, with the consent of the parents after they have been adequately informed, if the methods employed safeguard the life and integrity of the embryo and the mother, without subjecting them to disproportionate risks.[27] But this diagnosis is gravely opposed to

---

[27] The obligation to avoid disproportionate risks involves an authentic respect for human beings and the uprightness of therapeutic intentions. It implies that the doctor "above all... must carefully evaluate the possible negative consequences which the necessary use of a particular exploratory technique may have upon the unborn child and avoid recourse to diagnostic procedures which do not offer sufficient guarantees of their honest purpose and substantial harmlessness. And if, as often happens in human choices, a degree of risk must be undertaken, he will take care to assure that it is justified by a truly urgent need for the diagnosis and by the importance of the results that can be achieved by it for the benefit of the unborn child himself" (POPE JOHN PAUL II, *Discourse to Participants in the Pro-Life Movement Congress*, 3 December 1983: *Insegnamenti di Giovanni Paolo II*, V, 3 [1982] 1512). This clarification concerning "proportionate risk" is also to be kept in mind in the following sections of the present Instruction, whenever this term appears.

the moral law when it is done with the thought of possibly inducing an abortion depending upon the results: a diagnosis which shows the existence of a malformation or abnormality. The spouse or relatives or anyone else would similarly be acting in a manner contrary to the moral law if they were to counsel or impose such a diagnostic procedure on the expectant mother with the same intention of possibly proceeding to an abortion. So too the specialist would be guilty of illicit collaboration if, in conducting the diagnosis and in communicating its results, he were deliberately to contribute to establishing or favoring a link between prenatal diagnosis and abortion.

32. In conclusion, any directive or programme of the civil and health authorities or of scientific organizations which in any way were to favor a link between prenatal diagnosis and abortion, or which were to go as far as directly to induce expectant mothers to submit to prenatal diagnosis planned for the purpose of eliminating foetuses which are affected by malformations or which are carriers of hereditary illness, is to be condemned as a violation of the unborn child's right to life and as an abuse of the prior rights and duties of the spouses.

## 3. ARE THERAPEUTIC PROCEDURES CARRIED OUT ON THE HUMAN EMBRYO LICIT?

33. As with all medical interventions on patients, *one must uphold as licit procedures carried out on the human embryo which respect the life and integrity of the embryo and do not involve disproportionate risks for it but are directed towards its healing, the improvement of its condition of health, or its individual survival.*

34. Whatever the type of medical, surgical or other

therapy, the free and informed consent of the parents is required, according to the deontological rules followed in the case of children. The application of this moral principle may call for delicate and particular precautions in the case of embryonic or foetal life.

35. The legitimacy and criteria of such procedures have been clearly stated by Pope John Paul II: "A strictly therapeutic intervention whose explicit objective is the healing of various maladies such as those stemming from chromosomal defects will, in principle, be considered desirable, provided it is directed to the true promotion of the personal well-being of the individual without doing harm to his integrity or worsening his condition of life. Such an intervention would indeed fall within the logic of Christian moral tradition".[28]

## 4. HOW IS ONE TO EVALUATE MORALLY RESEARCH AND EXPERIMENTATION* ON THE HU-

---

[28] POPE JOHN PAUL II, *Discourse to the Participants in the 35th General Assembly of the World Medical Association,* 29 October 1983: AAS 76 (1984) 392.

* Since the terms "research" and "experimentation" are often used equivalently and ambiguously, it is deemed necessary to specify the exact meaning given them in this document.

1) By *research* is meant any inductive-deductive process which aims at promoting the systematic observation of a given phenomenon in the human field or at verifying a hypothesis arising from previous observations.

2) By *experimentation* is meant any research in which the human being (in the various stages of his existence: embryo, foetus, child or adult) represents the object through which or upon which one intends to verify the effect, at present unknown or not sufficiently known, of a given treatment (e.g. pharmacological, teratogenic, surgical, etc.)

36.   *Medical research must refrain from operations on live embryos, unless there is a moral certainty of not causing harm to the life or integrity of the unborn child and the mother, and on condition that the parents have given their free and informed consent to the procedure.* It follows that all research, even when limited to the simple observation of the embryo, would become illicit were it to involve risk to the embryo's physical integrity or life by reason of the methods used or the effects induced.

37.   As regards experimentation, and presupposing the general distinction between experimentation for purposes which are not directly therapeutic and experimentation which is clearly therapeutic for the subject himself, in the case in point one must also distinguish between experimentation carried out on embryos which are still alive and experimentation carried out on embryos which are dead. *If the embryos are living, whether viable or not, they must be respected just like any other human person; experimentation on embryos which is not directly therapeutic is illicit.*[29]

38.   No objective, even though noble in itself, such as a foreseeable advantage to science, to other human beings or to society, can in any way justify experimentation on living human embryos or foetuses, whether viable or not, either inside or outside the mother's womb.   The informed consent ordinarily required for clinical experimentation on

---

[29] Cf. POPE JOHN PAUL II, *Address to a Meeting of the Pontifical Academy of Sciences*, 23 October 1982: AAS 75 (1983) 37: "I condemn, in the most explicit and formal way, experimental manipulations of the human embryo, since the human being, from conception to death, cannot be exploited for any purpose whatsoever".

adults cannot be granted by the parents, who may not freely dispose of the physical integrity or life of the unborn child. Moreover, experimentation on embryos and foetuses always involves risk, and indeed in most cases it involves the certain expectation of harm to their physical integrity or even their death.

39.   To use human embryos or foetuses as the object or instrument of experimentation constitutes a crime against their dignity as human beings having a right to the same respect that is due to the child already born and to every human person.

40.   The *Charter of the Rights of the Family* published by the Holy See affirms:   "Respect for the dignity of the human being excludes all experimental manipulation or exploitation of the human embryo".[30]   The practice of keeping alive human embryos *in vivo* or *in vitro* for experimental or commercial purposes is totally opposed to human dignity.

41.   In the case of experimentation that is clearly therapeutic, namely, when it is a matter of experimental forms of therapy used for the benefit of the embryo itself in a final attempt to save its life, and in the absence of other reliable forms of therapy, recourse to drugs or procedures not yet fully tested can be licit.[31]

---

[30] HOLY SEE, *Charter of the Rights of the Family*, 4b: *L'Osservatore Romano*, 25 November 1983.

[31] Cf. POPE JOHN PAUL II, *Address to the Participants in the Convention of the Pro-Life Movement*, 3 December 1982: *Insegnamenti di Giovanni Paolo II*, V,3 (1982) 1511: "Any form of experimentation on the foetus that may damage its integrity or worsen its condition is unacceptable, except in the case of a final effort to save it from death". *SACRED CONGREGATION FOR THE DOCTRINE OF THE FAITH, Declaration on Euthanasia*, 4: AAS 72 (1980) 550: "In the absence of other sufficient remedies, it is permitted, with the

42.   *The corpses of human embryos and foetuses, whether they have been deliberately aborted or not, must be respected just as the remains of other human beings.* In particular, they cannot be subjected to mutilation or to autopsies if their death has not yet been verified and without the consent of the parents or of the mother.  Furthermore, the moral requirements must be safeguarded that there be no complicity in deliberate abortion and that the risk of scandal be avoided.  Also, in the case of dead foetuses, as for the corpses of adult persons, all commercial trafficking must be considered illicit and should be prohibited.

## 5. HOW IS ONE TO EVALUATE MORALLY THE USE FOR RESEARCH PURPOSES OF EMBRYOS OBTAINED BY FERTILIZATION "IN VITRO"?

43.   Human embryos obtained *in vitro* are human beings and subjects with rights:  their dignity and right to life must be respected from the first moment of their existence. *It is immoral to produce human embryos destined to be exploited as disposable "biological material."*

44.   In the usual practice of *in vitro* fertilization, not all of the embryos are transferred to the woman's body; some are destroyed.  Just as the Church condemns induced abortion, so she also forbids acts against the life of these human beings. *It is a duty to condemn the particular gravity of the voluntary destruction of human embryos obtained "in vitro" for the sole purpose of research, either by means of*

---

patients's consent, to have recourse to the means provided by the most advanced medical techniques, even if these means are still at the experimental stage and are not without a certain risk".

316

*artificial insemination or by means of "twin fission."* By acting in this way the researcher usurps the place of God; and, even though he may be unaware of this, he sets himself up as the master of the destiny of others inasmuch as he arbitrarily chooses whom he will allow to live and whom he will send to death and kills defenseless human beings.

45. Methods of observation or experimentation which damage or impose grave and disproportionate risks upon embryos obtained *in vitro* are morally illicit for the same reasons. Every human being is to be respected for himself, and cannot be reduced in worth to a pure and simple instrument for the advantage of others. *It is therefore not in conformity with the moral law deliberately to expose to death human embryos obtained "in vitro."* In consequence of the fact that they have been produced *in vitro*, those embryos which are not transferred into the body of the mother and are called "spare" are exposed to an absurd fate, with no possibility of their being offered safe means of survival which can be licitly pursued.

## 6. WHAT JUDGMENT SHOULD BE MADE ON OTHER PROCEDURES OF MANIPULATING EMBRYOS CONNECTED WITH THE "TECHNIQUES OF HUMAN REPRODUCTION"?

46. Techniques of fertilization *in vitro* can open the way to other forms of biological and genetic manipulation of human embryos, such as attempts or plans for fertilization between human and animal gametes and the gestation of human embryos in the uterus of animals, or the hypothesis or project of constructing artificial uteruses for the human embryo. *These procedures are contrary to the human*

*dignity proper to the embryo, and at the same time they are contrary to the right of every person to be conceived and to be born within marriage and from marriage.*[32] *Also, attempts or hypotheses for obtaining a human being without any connection with sexuality through "twin fission," cloning or parthenogenesis are to be considered contrary to the moral law, since they are in opposition to the dignity both of human procreation and of the conjugal union.*

47. *The freezing of embryos,* even when carried out in order to preserve the life of an embryo — cryopreservation — *constitutes an offense against the respect due to human beings* by exposing them to grave risks of death or harm to their physical integrity and depriving them, at least temporarily, of maternal shelter and gestation, thus placing them in a situation in which further offenses and manipulation are possible.

48. *Certain attempts to influence chromosomic or genetic inheritance are not therapeutic but are aimed at producing human beings selected according to sex or other predetermined qualities. These manipulations are contrary to the personal dignity of the human being and his or her integrity and identity.* Therefore in no way can they be justified on the grounds of possible beneficial consequences for future

---

[32] No one, before coming into existence, can claim a subjective right to begin to exist; nevertheless, it is legitimate to affirm the right of the child to have a fully human origin through conception in conformity with the personal nature of the human being. Life is a gift that must be bestowed in a manner worthy both of the subject receiving it and of the subjects transmitting it. This statement is to be borne in mind also for what will be explained concerning artificial human procreation.

humanity.[33]  Every person must be respected for himself: in this consists the dignity and right of every human being from his or her beginning.

## II
## INTERVENTIONS UPON HUMAN PROCREATION

49.  By "artificial procreation" or "artificial fertilization" are understood here the different technical procedures directed towards obtaining a human conception in a manner other than the sexual union of man and woman.  This Instruction deals with fertilization of an ovum in a test-tube (*in vitro* fertilization) and artificial insemination through transfer into the woman's genital tracts of previously collected sperm.

50.  A preliminary point for the moral evaluation of such technical procedures is constituted by the consideration of the circumstances and consequences which those procedures involve in relation to the respect due the human embryo. Development of the practice of *in vitro* fertilization has required innumerable fertilization and destructions of human embryos.  Even today, the usual practice presupposes a hyper-ovulation on the part of the woman: a number of ova are withdrawn fertilized and then cultivated *in vitro* for some days.  Usually not all are transferred into the genital tracts of the woman; some embryos, generally called "spare," are destroyed or frozen.  On occasion, some of the implanted embryos are sacrificed for various eugenic, eco-

---

[33] Cf. POPE JOHN PAUL II, *Discourse to those taking part in the 35th General Assembly of the World Medical Association*, 29 October 1983; AAS 76 (1984) 391.

nomic or psychological reasons. Such deliberate destruction of human beings or their utilization for different purposes to the detriment of their integrity and life is contrary to the doctrine on procured abortion already recalled.

51.    The connection between *in vitro* fertilization and the voluntary destruction of human embryos occurs too often. This is significant: through these procedures, with apparently contrary purposes, life and death are subjected to the decision of man, who thus sets himself up as the giver of life and death by decree. This dynamic of violence and domination may remain unnoticed by those very individuals who, in wishing to utilize this procedure, become subject to it themselves. The facts recorded and the cold logic which links them must be taken into consideration for a moral judgment on IVF and ET (*in vitro* fertilization and embryo transfer): the abortion-mentality which has made this procedure possible thus leads, whether one wants it or not, to man's domination over the life and death of his fellow human beings and can lead to a system of radical eugenics.

52.    Nevertheless, such abuses do not exempt one from a further and thorough ethical study of the techniques of artificial procreation considered in themselves, abstracting as far as possible from the destruction of embryos produced *in vitro*.

53.    The present Instruction will therefore take into consideration in the first place the problems posed by heterologous artificial fertilization (II, 1-3),* and subse-

---

* By the term *heterologous artificial fertilization* or *procreation*, the Instruction means techniques used to obtain a human conception artificially by the use of gametes coming from at least one donor other than the spouses who are joined in marriage. Such techniques can be of two types:

   a) *Heterologous IVF and ET*: the technique used to obtain a human conception through the meeting *in vitro* of gametes taken from at least one

quently those linked with homologous artificial fertilization (II, 4-6).**

54. Before formulating an ethical judgment on each of these procedures, the principles and values which determine the moral evaluation of each of them will be considered.

# A
# HETEROLOGOUS ARTIFICIAL FERTILIZATION

## 1. WHY MUST HUMAN PROCREATION TAKE PLACE IN MARRIAGE?

55. *Every human being is always to be accepted as a gift and blessing of God. However, from the moral point of view a truly responsible procreation vis-à-vis the unborn child must be the fruit of marriage.*

56. For human procreation has specific characteristics by

---

donor other than the two spouses joined in marriage.

b) *Heterologous artificial insemination:* the technique used to obtain a human conception through the transfer into the genital tracts of the woman of the sperm previously collected from a donor other than the husband.

** By *artificial homologous fertilization or procreation*, the Instruction means the technique used to obtain a human conception using the gametes of the two spouses joined in marriage. Homologous artificial fertilization can be carried out by two different methods:

a) *Homologous IVF and ET:* the technique used to obtain a human conception through the meeting *in vitro* of the gametes of the spouses joined in marriage.

b) *Homologous artificial insemination:* the technique used to obtain a human conception through the transfer into the genital tracts of a married woman of the sperm previously collected from her husband.

and the woman collaborate with the power of the Creator, must be the fruit and the sign of the mutual self-giving of the spouses, of their love and of their fidelity.[34] *The fidelity of the spouses in the unity of marriage involves reciprocal respect of their right to become a father and a mother only through each other.*

57. The child has the right to be conceived, carried in the womb, brought into the world and brought up within marriage: it is through the secure and recognized relationship to his own parents that the child can discover his own identity and achieve his own proper human development.

58. The parents find in their child a confirmation and completion of their reciprocal self-giving: the child is the living image of their love, the permanent sign of their conjugal union, the living and indissoluble concrete expression of their paternity and maternity.[35]

59. By reason of the vocation and social responsibilities of the person, the good of the children and of the parents contributes to the good of civil society; the vitality and stability of society require that children come into the world within a family and that the family be firmly based on marriage.

60. The tradition of the Church and anthropological reflection recognize in marriage and in its indissoluble unity the only setting worthy of truly responsible procreation.

---

[34] Cf. Pastoral Constitution on the Church in the Modern World, *Gaudium et Spes*, 50.

[35] Cf. POPE JOHN PAUL II, Apostolic Exhortation *Familiaris Consortio*, 14: AAS 74 (1982) 96.

## 2. DOES HETEROLOGOUS ARTIFICIAL FERTILIZATION CONFORM TO THE DIGNITY OF THE COUPLE AND TO THE TRUTH OF MARRIAGE?

61. Through IVF and ET and heterologous artificial insemination, human conception is achieved through the fusion of gametes of at least one donor other than the spouses who are united in marriage. *Heterologous artificial fertilization is contrary to the unity of marriage, to the dignity of the spouses, to the vocation proper to parents, and to the child's right to be conceived and brought into the world in marriage and from marriage.*[36]

62. Respect for the unity of marriage and for conjugal fidelity demands that the child be conceived in marriage; the bond existing between husband and wife accords the spouses, in an objective and inalienable manner, the exclusive right to become father and mother solely through

---

[36] Cf. POPE PIUS XII, *Discourse to those taking part in the 4th International Congress of Catholic Doctors*, 29 September 1949: AAS 41 (1949) 559. According to the plan of the Creator, "A man leaves his father and his mother and cleaves to his wife, and they become one flesh" (*Gen* 2:24). The unity of marriage, bound to the order of creation, is a truth accessible to natural reason. The Church's Tradition and Magisterium frequently make reference to the Book of Genesis, both directly and through the passages of the New Testament that refer to it: *Mt* 19:4-6; *Mk* 10:5-8; *Eph* 5:31. Cf. ATHENAGORAS, *Legatio pro christianis*, 33: *PG* 6, 965-967; ST CHRYSOSTOM, *In Matthaeum homiliae*, LXII, 19, 1: *PG* 58 597; ST LEO THE GREAT, *Epist. ad Rusticum*, 4: *PL* 54, 1204; INNOCENT III, Epist. *Gaudemus in Domino*: *DS* 778; COUNCIL OF LYONS II, *IV Session*: *DS* 860; COUNCIL OF TRENT, XXIV *Session*: *DS* 1798. 1802; POPE LEO XIII, Encyclical *Arcanum Divinae Sapientiae;* ASS 12 (1879/80) 338-391; POPE PIUS XI, Encyclical *Casti Connubii*: AAS 74 (1982) 101-102; *Code of Canon Law*, Can. 1056.

each other.[37]   Recourse to the gametes of a third person, in order to have sperm or ovum available, constitutes a violation of the reciprocal commitment of the spouses and a grave lack in regard to that essential property of marriage which is its unity.

63.   Heterologous artificial fertilization violates the rights of the child; it deprives him of his filial relationship with his parental origins and can hinder the maturing of his personal identity.   Furthermore, it offends the common vocation of the spouses who are called to fatherhood and motherhood: it objectively deprives conjugal fruitfulness of its unity and integrity; it brings about and manifests a rupture between genetic parenthood, gestational parenthood and responsibility for upbringing.   Such damage to the personal relationship within the family has repercussions on civil society: what threatens the unity and stability of the family is a source of dissension, disorder and injustice in the whole of social life.

64.   *These reasons lead to a negative moral judgment concerning heterologous artificial fertilization: consequently fertilization of a married woman with the sperm of a donor different from her husband and fertilization with the husband's sperm of an ovum not coming from his wife are morally illicit.  Furthermore, the artificial fertilization of a woman who is unmarried or a widow, whoever the donor may be, cannot be morally justified.*

65.   The desire to have a child and the love between

---

[37] Cf. POPE PIUS XII, *Discourse to those taking part in the 4th International Congress of Catholic Doctors*, 29 September 1949: AAS 41 (1949) 560; *Discourse to those taking part in the Congress of the Italian Catholic Union of Midwives*, 29 October 1951: AAS 43 (1951) 850; *Code of Canon Law*, Can. 1134.

spouses who long to obviate a sterility which cannot be overcome in any other way constitute understandable motivations; but subjectively good intentions do not render heterologous artificial fertilization conformable to the objective and inalienable properties of marriage or respectful of the rights of the child and of the spouses.

## 3. IS "SURROGATE"* MOTHERHOOD MORALLY LICIT?

66. No, *for the same reasons which lead one to reject heterologous artificial fertilization: for it is contrary to the unity of marriage and to the dignity of the procreation of the human person.*

67. Surrogate motherhood represents an objective failure to meet the obligations of maternal love, of conjugal fidelity and of responsible motherhood; it offends the dignity and the right of the child to be conceived, carried in the womb, brought into the world and brought up by his own parents; it sets up, to the detriment of families, a division between the physical, psychological and moral elements which constitute those families.

---

* By "surrogate mother" the Instruction means:

a) the woman who carries in pregnancy an embryo implanted in her uterus and who is genetically a stranger to the embryo because it has been obtained through the union of the gametes of "donors." She carries the pregnancy with a pledge to surrender the baby once it is born to the party who commissioned or made the agreement for the pregnancy.

b) the woman who carries in pregnancy an embryo to whose procreation she has contributed the donation of her own ovum, fertilized through insemination with the sperm of a man other than her husband. She carries the pregnancy with a pledge to surrender the child once it is born to the party who commissioned or made the agreement for the pregnancy.

# B
## HOMOLOGOUS ARTIFICIAL FERTILIZATION

68. Since heterologous artificial fertilization has been declared unacceptable, the question arises of how to evaluate morally the process of homologous artificial fertilization: IVF and ET and artificial insemination between husband and wife. First a question of principle must be clarified.

## 4. WHAT CONNECTION IS REQUIRED FROM THE MORAL POINT OF VIEW BETWEEN PROCREATION AND THE CONJUGAL ACT?

69. a) The Church's teaching on marriage and human procreation affirms the "inseparable connection, willed by God and unable to be broken by man on his own initiative, between the two meanings of the conjugal act: the unitive meaning and the procreative meaning. Indeed, by its intimate structure, the conjugal act, while most closely uniting husband and wife, capacitates them for the generation of new lives, according to laws inscribed in the very being of man and of woman".[38] This principle, which is based upon the nature of marriage and the intimate connection of the goods of marriage, has well-known consequences on the level of responsible fatherhood and motherhood. "By safeguarding both these essential aspects, the unitive and the procreative, the conjugal act preserves in its fullness the sense of true mutual love and its ordination

---

[38] POPE PAUL VI, Encyclical Letter *Humanae Vitae*, 12; AAS 60 (1968) 488-489.

towards man's exalted vocation to parenthood."[39]

70. The same doctrine concerning the link between the meanings of conjugal act and between the goods of marriage throws light on the moral problem of homologous artificial fertilization, since "it is never permitted to separate these different aspects to such a degree as positively to exclude either the procreative intention or the conjugal relation."[40]

71. Contraception deliberately deprives the conjugal act of its openness to procreation and in this way brings about a voluntary dissociation of the ends of marriage. Homologous artificial fertilization, in seeking a procreation which is not the fruit of a specific act of conjugal union, objectively effects an analogous separation between the goods and the meanings of marriage.

72. Thus, *fertilization is licitly sought when it is the result of a "conjugal act which is per se suitable for the generation of children to which marriage is ordered by its nature and by which the spouses become one flesh."[41] But from the moral point of view procreation is deprived of its proper perfection when it is not desired as the fruit of the conjugal act, that is to say of the specific act of the spouses' union.*

73. b) The moral value of the intimate link between the

---

[39] *Loc. cit., ibid.,* 489.

[40] POPE PIUS XII, *Discourse to those taking part in the Second Naples World Congress on Fertility and Human Sterility,* 19 May 1956: AAS 48 (1956) 470.

[41] *Code of Canon Law,* Can. 1061. According to this Canon, the conjugal act is that by which the marriage is consummated if the couple "have performed (it) between themselves in a human manner."

goods of marriage and between the meanings of the conjugal act is based upon the unity of the human being, a unity involving body and spiritual soul.[42] Spouses mutually express their personal love in the "language of the body," which clearly involves both "sponsal meanings" and parental ones.[43] The conjugal act by which the couple mutually express their self-gift at the same time expresses openness to the gift of life. It is an act that is inseparably corporal and spiritual. It is in their bodies and through their bodies that the spouses consummate their marriage and are able to become father and mother. In order to respect the language of their bodies and their natural generosity, the conjugal union must take place with respect for its openness to procreation; and the procreation of a person must be the fruit and the result of married love. The origin of the human being thus follows from a procreation that is "linked to the union, not only biological but also spiritual, of the parents, made one by the bond of marriage."[44] Fertilization achieved outside the bodies of the couple remains by this very fact deprived of the meanings and the values which are expressed in the language of the body and in the union of human persons.

74. c) Only respect for the link between the meanings of the conjugal act and respect for the unity of the human

---

[42] Cf. Pastoral Constitution *Gaudium et Spes*, 14.

[43] Cf. POPE JOHN PAUL II, *General Audience on 16 January 1980*: *Insegnamenti di Giovanni Paolo I*, III, 1 (1980) 148-152.

[44] POPE JOHN PAUL II, *Discourse to those taking part in the 35th General Assembly of the World Medical Association*, 29 October 1983: AAS 76 (1984) 393.

being make possible procreation in conformity with the dignity of the person. In his unique and irrepeatable origin, the child must be respected and recognized as equal in personal dignity to those who give him life. The human person must be accepted in his parents' act of union and love; the generation of a child must therefore be the fruit of that mutual giving[45] which is realized in the conjugal act wherein the spouses cooperate as servants and not as masters in the work of the Creator who is Love.[46]

75.  In reality, the origin of a human person is the result of an act of giving. The one conceived must be the fruit of his parents' love. He cannot be desired or conceived as the product of an intervention of medical or biological techniques; that would be equivalent to reducing him to an object of scientific technology. No one may subject the coming of a child into the world to conditions of technical efficiency which are to be evaluated according to standards of control and dominion.

76.  *The moral relevance of the link between the meanings of the conjugal act and between the goods of marriage, as well as the unity of the human being and the dignity of his origin, demand that the procreation of a human person be brought about as the fruit of the conjugal act specific to the love between spouses.* The link between procreation and the conjugal act is thus shown to be of great importance on the anthropological and moral planes, and it throws light on the position of the Magisterium with regard to homologous artificial fertilization.

---

[45] Cf. Pastoral Constitution *Gaudium et Spes*, 51.

[46] Cf. Pastoral Constitution *Gaudium et Spes*, 50.

## 5.  IS HOMOLOGOUS "IN VITRO" FERTILIZATION MORALLY LICIT?

77.   The answer to this question is strictly dependent on the principles just mentioned.  Certainly one cannot ignore the legitimate aspirations of sterile couples.  For some, recourse to homologous IVF and ET appears to be the only way of fulfilling their sincere desire for a child.  The question is asked whether the totality of conjugal life in such situations is not sufficient to ensure the dignity proper to human procreation.  It is acknowledged that IVF and ET certainly cannot supply for the absence of sexual relations[47] and cannot be preferred to the specific acts of conjugal union, given the risks involved for the child and the difficulties of the procedure.  but it is asked whether, when there is no other way of overcoming the sterility which is a source of suffering, homologous *in vitro* fertilization may not constitute an aid, if not a form of therapy, whereby its moral licitness could be admitted.

78.   The desire for a child — or at the very least an openness to the transmission of life — is a necessary prerequisite from the moral point of view for responsible human procreation.  but this good intention is not sufficient for making a positive moral evaluation of *in vitro* fertilization between spouses.  The process of IVF and ET must be judged in itself and cannot borrow its definitive moral quality from the totality of conjugal life of which it be-

---

[47] Cf. POPE PIUS XII, *Discourse to those taking part in the 4th International Congress of Catholic Doctors*, 29 September 1949:  AAS 41 (1949) 560:  "It would be erroneous... to think that the possibility of resorting to this means (artificial fertilization) might render valid a marrige between persons unable to contract it because of the *impedimentum impotentiae*".

comes part nor from the conjugal acts which may precede or follow it.[48]

79. It has already been recalled that, in the circumstances in which it is regularly practiced, IVF and ET involves the destruction of human beings, which is something contrary to the doctrine on the illicitness of abortion previously mentioned.[49] But even in a situation in which every precaution were taken to avoid the death of human embryos, homologous IVF and ET dissociates from the conjugal act the actions which are directed to human fertilization. For this reason the very nature of homologous IVF and ET also must be taken into account, even abstracting from the link with procured abortion.

80. Homologous IVF and ET is brought about outside the bodies of the couple through actions of third parties whose competence and technical activity determine the success of the procedure. Such fertilization entrusts the life and identity of the embryo into the power of doctors and biologists and establishes the domination of technology over the origin and destiny of the human person. Such a relationship of domination is in itself contrary to the dignity and equality that must be common to parents and children.

81. Conception *in vitro* is the result of the technical action which presides over fertilization. *Such fertilization is neither in fact achieved nor positively willed as the expression and fruit of a specific act of the conjugal union. In homologous IVF and ET, therefore, even if it is considered*

---

[48] A similar question was dealt with by POPE PAUL VI, Encyclical *Humanae Vitae*, 14: AAS 60 (1968) 490-491.

[49] Cf. *supra*: I, 1 ff.

*in the context of "de facto" existing sexual relations, the generation of the human person is objectively deprived of its proper perfection: namely, that of being the result and fruit of a conjugal act* in which the spouses can become "cooperators with God for giving life to a new person".[50]

82.  These reasons enable us to understand why the act of conjugal love is considered in the teaching of the Church as the only setting worthy of human procreation.  For the same reasons the so-called "simple case," i.e. a homologous IVF and ET procedure that is free of any compromise with the abortive practice of destroying embryos and with masturbation, remains a technique which is morally illicit because it deprives human procreation of the dignity which is proper and connatural to it.

83.  Certainly, homologous IVF and ET fertilization is not marked by all that ethical negativity found in extra-conjugal procreation; the family and marriage continue to constitute the setting for the birth and upbringing of the children. Nevertheless, in conformity with the traditional doctrine relating to the goods of marriage and the dignity of the person, *the Church remains opposed from the moral point of view to homologous "in vitro" fertilization.  Such fertilization is in itself illicit and in opposition to the dignity of procreation and of the conjugal union, even when everything is done to avoid the death of the human embryo.*

84.  Although the manner in which human conception is achieved with IVF and ET cannot be approved, every child which comes into the world must in any case be accepted as a living gift of the divine Goodness and must be brought

---

[50] POPE JOHN PAUL II, Apostolic Exhortation *Familiaris Consortio*, 14: AAS 74 (1982) 96.

up with love.

## 6. HOW IS HOMOLOGOUS ARTIFICIAL INSEMINATION TO BE EVALUATED FROM THE MORAL POINT OF VIEW?

85.  *Homologous artificial insemination within marriage cannot be admitted except for those cases in which the technical means is not a substitute for the conjugal act but serves to facilitate and to help so that the act attains its natural purpose.*

86.  The teaching of the Magisterium on this point has already been stated.[51] This teaching is not just an expression of particular historical circumstances but is based on the Church's doctrine concerning the connection between the conjugal union and procreation and on a consideration of the personal nature of the conjugal act and of human procreation. "In its natural structure, the conjugal act is a personal action, a simultaneous and immediate cooperation on the part of the husband and wife, which by the very nature of the agents and the proper nature of the act is the expression of the mutual gift which, according to the words

---

[51] Cf. *Response of the Holy Office*, 17 March 1897: DS 3323; POPE PIUS XII, *Discourse to those taking part in the 4th International Congress of Catholic Doctors*, 29 September 1949: AAS 41 (1949) 560; *Discourse to the Italian Catholic Union of Midwives*, 29 October 1951: AAS 43 (1951) 850; *Discourse to those taking part in the Second Naples World Congress on Fertility and Human Sterility*, 19 May 1956: AAS 48 (1956) 471-473; *Discourse to those taking part in the 7th International Congress of the International Society of Haematology*, 12 September 1958: AAS 50 (1958) 733; POPE JOHN XXIII, Encyclical *Mater et Magistra*, III: AAS 53 (1961) 447.

of Scripture, brings about union 'in one flesh.'"[52] Thus moral conscience "does not necessarily proscribe the use of certain artificial means destined solely either to the facilitating of the natural act or to ensuring that the natural act normally performed achieves its proper end".[53] If the technical means facilitates the conjugal act or helps it to reach its natural objectives, it can be morally acceptable. If, on the other hand, the procedure were to replace the conjugal act, it is morally illicit.

87.   Artificial insemination as a substitute for the conjugal act is prohibited by reason of the voluntarily achieved dissociation of the two meanings of the conjugal act. Masturbation, through which the sperm is normally obtained, is another sign of this dissociation: even when it is done for the purpose of procreation, the act remains deprived of its unitive meaning:   "It lacks the sexual relationship called for by the moral order, namely the relationship which realizes 'the full sense of mutual self-giving and human procreation in the context of true love.'"[54]

---

[52] POPE PIUS XII, *Discourse to the Italian Catholic Union of Midwives*, 29 October 1951:  AAS 43 (1951) 850.

[53] POPE PIUS XII, *Discourse to those taking part in the 4th International Congress of Catholic Doctors*, 29 September 1949:  AAS 41 (1949) 560.

[54] SACRED CONGREGATION FOR THE DOCTRINE OF THE FAITH, *Declaration on Certain Questions Concerning Sexual Ethics*, 9: AAS 68, *which quotes the Pastoral Constitution Gaudium et Spes*, 51. Cf. *Decree of the Holy Office*, 2 August 1929: AAS 21 (1929) 490; POPE PIUS XII, *Discourse to those taking part in the 26th Congress of the Italian Society of Urology*, 8 October 1953: AAS 45 (1953) 678.

## 7.  WHAT MORAL CRITERION CAN BE PROPOSED WITH REGARD TO MEDICAL INTERVENTION IN HUMAN PROCREATION?

88.  The medical act must be evaluated not only with reference to its technical dimension but also and above all in relation to its goal which is the good of persons and their bodily and psychological health.  The moral criteria for medical intervention in procreation are deduced from the dignity of human persons, of their sexuality and of their origin.

89.  *Medicine which seeks to be ordered to the integral good of the person must respect the specifically human values of sexuality.*[55]  *The doctor is at the service of persons and of human procreation.  He does not have the authority to dispose of them or to decide their fate.*  A medical intervention respects the dignity of persons when it seeks to assist the conjugal act either in order to facilitate its performance or in order to enable it to achieve its objective once it has been normally performed".[56]

90.  On the other hand, it sometimes happens that a medical procedure technologically replaces the conjugal act in order to obtain a procreation which is neither its result nor its fruit.  In this case the medical act is not, as it should be, at the service of conjugal union but rather appropriates to itself the procreative function and thus contradicts the dignity and the inalienable rights of the spouses and of the

---

[55] Cf. POPE JOHN XXIII, Encyclical *Mater et magistra*, III:  AAS 53 (1961) 447.

[56] Cf. POPE PIUS XII, *Discourse to those taking part in the 4th International Congress of Catholic Doctors*, 29 September 1949:  AAS 41 (1949), 560.

child to be born.

91.   The humanization of medicine, which is insisted upon today by everyone, requires respect for the integral dignity of the human person first of all in the act and at the moment in which the spouses transmit life to a new person. It is only logical therefore to address an urgent appeal to Catholic doctors and scientists that they bear exemplary witness to the respect due to the human embryo and to the dignity of procreation.   The medical and nursing staff of Catholic hospitals and clinics are in a special way urged to do justice to the moral obligations which they have assumed, frequently also, as part of their contract.   Those who are in charge of Catholic hospitals and clinics and who are often Religious will take special care to safeguard and promote a diligent observance of the moral norms recalled in the present Instruction.

## 8.   THE SUFFERING CAUSED BY INFERTILITY IN MARRIAGE

92.   *The suffering of spouses who cannot have children or who are afraid of bringing a handicapped child into the world is a suffering that everyone must understand and properly evaluate.*

93.   On the part of the spouses, the desire for a child is natural:   it expresses the vocation to fatherhood and motherhood inscribed in conjugal love.  This desire can be even stronger if the couple is affected by sterility which appears incurable.  Nevertheless, marriage does not confer upon the spouses the right to have a child, but only the right to perform those natural acts which are *per se* ordered

to procreation.[57]

94.  *A true and proper right to a child would be contrary to the child's dignity and nature. The child is not an object to which one has a right, nor can he be considered as an object of ownership: rather, a child is a gift, "the supreme gift"[58] and the most gratuitous gift of marriage, and is a living testimony of the mutual giving of his parents. For this reason, the child has the right, as already mentioned, to be the fruit of the specific act of the conjugal love of his parents; and he also has the right to be respected as a person from the moment of his conception.*

95.  Nevertheless, whatever its cause or prognosis, sterility is certainly a difficult trial. The community of believers is called to shed light upon and support the suffering of those who are unable to fulfill their legitimate aspiration to motherhood and fatherhood. Spouses who find themselves in this sad situation are called to find in it an opportunity for sharing in a particular way in the Lord's Cross, the source of spiritual fruitfulness. Sterile couples must not forget that "even when procreation is not possible, conjugal life does not for this reason lose its value. Physical sterility in fact can be for spouses the occasion for other important services to the life of the human person, for example, adoption, various forms of educational work, and assistance

---

[57] Cf. POPE PIUS XII, *Discourse to those taking part in the Second Naples World Congress on Fertility and Human Sterility*, 19 May 1956:  AAS 48 (1956) 471-473.

[58] Pastoral Constitution *Gaudium et Spes*, 50.

to other families and to poor or handicapped children".[59]

96.  Many researchers are engaged in the fight against sterility.  While fully safeguarding the dignity of human procreation, some have achieved results which previously seemed unattainable.  Scientists therefore are to be encouraged to continue their research with the aim of preventing the causes of sterility and of being able to remedy them so that sterile couples will be able to procreate in full respect for their own personal dignity and that of the child to be born.

## III
## MORAL AND CIVIL LAW

## THE VALUES AND MORAL OBLIGATIONS
## THAT CIVIL LEGISLATION
## MUST RESPECT AND SANCTION IN THIS MATTER

97.  The inviolable right to life of every innocent human individual and the rights of the family and of the institution of marriage constitute fundamental moral values, because they concern the natural condition and integral vocation of the human person; at the same time they are constitutive elements of civil society and its order.

98.  For this reason the new technological possibilities which have opened up in the field of biomedicine require the intervention of the political authorities and of the legislator, since an uncontrolled application of such techniques could lead to unforeseeable and damaging consequences for civil society.  Recourse to the conscience of

---

[59] POPE JOHN PAUL II, Apostolic Exhortation *Familiaris Consortio*, 14:  AAS 74 (1982) 97.

each individual and to the self-regulation of researchers cannot be sufficient for ensuring respect for personal rights and public order. If the legislator responsible for the common good were not watchful, he could be deprived of his prerogatives by researchers claiming to govern humanity in the name of the biological discoveries and the alleged "improvement" processes which they would draw from those discoveries. "Eugenism" and forms of discrimination between human beings could come to be legitimized: this would constitute an act of violence and a serious offense to the equality, dignity and fundamental rights of the human person.

99. The intervention of the public authority must be inspired by the rational principles which regulate the relationships between civil law and moral law. The task of the civil law is to ensure the common good of people through the recognition of and the defense of fundamental rights and through the promotion of peace and of public morality.[60] In no sphere of life can the civil law take the place of conscience or dictate norms concerning things which are outside its competence. It must sometimes tolerate, for the sake of public order, things which it cannot forbid without a greater evil resulting. However, the inalienable rights of the person must be recognized and respected by civil society and the political authority. These human rights depend neither on single individuals nor on parents; nor do they represent a concession made by society and the State: they pertain to human nature and are inherent in the person by virtue of the creative act from which the person took his or her origin.

---

[60] Cf. Declaration *Dignitatis Humanae*, 7.

100. Among such fundamental rights one should mention in this regard: a) every human being's right to life and physical integrity from the moment of conception until death; b) the rights of the family and of marriage as an institution and, in this area, the child's right to be conceived, brought into the world and brought up by his parents. To each of these two themes it is necessary here to give some further consideration.

101. In various States certain laws have authorized the direct suppression of innocents: the moment a positive law deprives a category of human beings of the protection which civil legislation must accord them, the State is denying the equality of all before law. When the State does not place its power at the service of the rights of each citizen, and in particular of the more vulnerable, the very foundations of a State based on law are undermined. The political authority consequently cannot give approval to the calling of human beings into existence through procedures which would expose them to those very grave risks noted previously. The possible recognition by positive law and the political authorities of techniques of artificial transmission of life and the experimentation connected with it would widen the breach already opened by the legalization of abortion.

102. As a consequence of the respect and protection which must be ensured for the unborn child from the moment of his conception, the law must provide appropriate penal sanctions for every deliberate violation of the child's rights. The law cannot tolerate — indeed it must expressly forbid — that human beings, even at the embryonic stage, should be treated as objects of experimentation, be mutilated or destroyed with the excuse that they are superfluous or incapable of developing normally.

103. The political authority is bound to guarantee to the institution of the family, upon which society is based, the juridical protection to which it has a right. From the very fact that it is at the service of people, the political authority must also be at the service of the family. Civil law cannot grant approval to techniques of artificial procreation which, for the benefit of third parties (doctors, biologists, economic or governmental powers), take away what is a right inherent in the relationship between spouses; and therefore civil law cannot legalize the donation of gametes between persons who are not legitimately united in marriage.

104. Legislation must also prohibit, by virtue of the support which is due to the family, embryo banks, *post mortem* insemination and "surrogate motherhood."

105. *It is part of the duty of the public authority to ensure that the civil law is regulated according to the fundamental norms of the moral law in matters concerning human rights, human life and the institution of the family. Politicians must commit themselves, through their interventions upon public opinion, to securing in society the widest possible consensus on such essential points and to consolidating this consensus wherever it risks being weakened or is in danger of collapse.*

106. In many countries, the legalization of abortion and juridical tolerance of unmarried couples makes it more difficult to secure respect for the fundamental rights recalled by this Instruction. It is to be hoped that States will not become responsible for aggravating these socially damaging situations of injustice. It is rather to be hoped that nations and States will realize all the cultural, ideological and political implications connected with the techniques of artificial procreation and will find the wisdom and courage necessary for issuing laws which are more just and

more respectful of human life and the institution of the family.

107. *The civil legislation of many states confers an undue legitimation upon certain practices in the eyes of many today; it is seen to be incapable of guaranteeing that morality which is in conformity with the natural exigencies of the human person and with the "unwritten laws" etched by the Creator upon the human heart. All men of good will must commit themselves, particularly within their professional field and in the exercise of their civil rights, to ensuring the reform of morally unacceptable civil laws and the correction of illicit practices. In addition, "conscientious objection" vis-a-vis such laws must be supported and recognized. A movement of passive resistance to the legitimation of practices contrary to human life and dignity is beginning to make an ever sharper impression upon the moral conscience of many, especially among specialists in the biomedical sciences.*

## CONCLUSION

108. The spread of technologies of intervention in the processes of human procreation raises very serious moral problems in relation to the respect due to the human being from the moment of conception, to the dignity of the person, of his or her sexuality, and of the transmission of life.

109. With this Instruction the Congregation for the Doctrine of the Faith, in fulfilling its responsibility to promote and defend the Church's teaching in so serious a matter, addresses a new and heartfelt invitation to all those who, by reason of their role and their commitment, can exercise a positive influence and ensure that, in the family and in society, due respect is accorded to life and love. It address-

es this invitation to those responsible for the formation of conscience and of public opinion, to scientists and medical professionals, to jurists and politicians. It hopes that all will understand the incompatibility between recognition of the dignity of the human person and contempt for life and love, between faith in the living God and the claim to decide arbitrarily the origin and fate of a human being.

110. In particular, the Congregation for the Doctrine of the Faith addresses an invitation with confidence and encouragement to theologians, and above all to moralists, that they study more deeply and make ever more accessible to the faithful the contents of the teaching of the Church's Magisterium in the light of a valid anthropology in the matter of sexuality and marriage and in the context of the necessary interdisciplinary approach. Thus they will make it possible to understand ever more clearly the reasons for and the validity of this teaching. By defending man against the excesses of his own power, the Church of God reminds him of the reasons for his true nobility; only in this way can the possibility of living and loving with that dignity and liberty which derive from respect for the truth be ensured for the men and women of tomorrow. The precise indication which are offered in the present Instruction therefore are not meant to halt the effort to reflection but rather to give it a renewed impulse in unrenounceable fidelity to the teaching of the Church.

111. In the light of the truth about the gift of human life and in the light of the moral principles which flow from that truth, everyone is invited to act in the area of responsibility proper to each and, like the good Samaritan, to recognize as a neighbor even the littlest among the children of men (Cf. *Lk* 10:29-37). Here Christ's words find a new and particular echo: "What you do to one of the least of my brethren, you do unto me" (*Mt* 25:40).

343

112. *During an audience granted to the undersigned Prefect after the plenary session of the Congregation for the Doctrine of the Faith, the Supreme Pontiff, John Paul II, approved this Instruction and ordered it to be published.* 113. Given at Rome, from the Congregation for the Doctrine of the Faith, February 22, 1987, the Feast of the Chair of St. Peter, the Apostle.

Joseph Card. Ratzinger
*Prefect*
Alberto Bovone
Titular Archbishop of Caesarea in Numidia
Secretary

# APPENDIX II

The following are the passages on morality and law from the *Declaration on Procured Abortion* of the Congregation for the Doctrine of the Faith. The translated text is from Austin Flannery, *ed.*, *Vatican Council II: More Postconciliar Documents*, pp. 447-449.

19. The moral discussion is being accompanied more or less everywhere by serious juridical debates. There is no country where legislation does not forbid and punish murder. Furthermore, many countries had specifically applied this condemnation and these penalties to the particular case of procured abortion. In these days a vast body of opinion petitions the liberalization of this latter prohibition. There already exists a fairly general tendency which seeks to limit as far as possible all restrictive legislation, especially when it seems to touch upon private life. The argument of pluralism is also used. Although many citizens — the argument goes — in particular the Catholic faithful, condemn abortion, many others hold that it is licit at least as a lesser evil. Why force them to follow an opinion which is not theirs, especially in a country where they are in the majority? In addition it is apparent that, where they still exist, the laws condemning abortion appear difficult to apply. The crime has become too common for it to be punished every time, and the public authorities often find that it is wiser to close their eyes to it. But the preservation of a law which is not applied is always to the detriment of authority and of all the other laws. It must be added that clandestine abortion seriously endangers the fertility and even the lives of women who resort to it. Even if the legislator continues to regard abortion as an evil, may he not propose to restrict its damage?

20. These arguments and others in addition that are heard from varying quarters are not conclusive. It is true that

civil law cannot expect to cover the whole field of morality or to punish all faults. No one expects it to do so. It must often tolerate what is in fact a lesser evil, in order to avoid a greater one. One must, however, be attentive to what a change in legislation can represent. Many will take as authorization what is perhaps only a refusal to punish. Even more, in the present case, this very refusal seems at the very least to admit that the legislator no longer considers abortion a crime against human life, since murder is still always severely punished. It is true that it is not the task of the law to choose between points of view or to impose one rather than another. But the life of the child takes precedence over all opinions. One cannot invoke freedom of thought to destroy life.

21. The role of law is not to record what is done, but to help in promoting improvement. It is at all times the task of the State to preserve each person's rights and to protect the weakest. In order to do so the State will have to right many wrongs. The law is not obliged to sanction everything, but it cannot act contrary to a law which is deeper and more majestic than any human law: the natural law engraved in men's hearts by the creator as a norm which reason clarifies and strives to formulate properly, and which one must always try to understand better, but which it is always wrong to contradict. Human law can abstain from punishment, but it cannot declare to be right what would be opposed to the natural law, for this opposition suffices to give the assurance that a law is not a law at all.

22. It must in any case be clearly understood that a Christian can never conform to a law which is in itself immoral, and such is the case of a law which would admit in principle the liceity of abortion. Nor can a Christian take part in a propaganda campaign in favor of such a law, or vote for it. Moreover, he may not collaborate in its

348

application. It is, for instance, inadmissible that doctors or nurses should find themselves obliged to cooperate closely in abortions and have to choose between the Christian law and their professional situation.

23. On the contrary it is the task of law to pursue a reform of society and of conditions of life in all milieux, starting with the most deprived, so that always and everywhere it may be possible to give every child coming into this world a welcome worthy of a person. Help for families and for unmarried mothers, assured grants for children, legislation for illegitimate children and reasonable arrangements for adoption — a whole positive policy must be put into force so that there will always be a concrete honorable and possible alternative to abortion.

# GLOSSARY OF TERMS

# GLOSSARY OF TERMS

**Abortion**: The word is used differently in medical and moral contexts. (The definitions given here are based on Thomas J O'Donnell, *Medicine and Christian Morality*, Alba House, 1976, pp. 137-144.)

1) *Medical*: The removal of a non-viable fetus from the uterus; or the killing and removal of a viable fetus. a) *Induced abortion*: An abortion which is brought about intentionally. b) *Spontaneous abortion*: A miscarriage; the accidental loss of the unborn child. Induced abortion is also considered as therapeutic or criminal. a) *Therapeutic abortion*: An abortion performed purposely, with the intent to save the life of the mother or to preserve her physical or mental health. b) *Criminal abortion*: An abortion performed purposely and in violation of the civil law.

2) *Moral*: The killing and removal of a fetus, viable or non-viable, from the uterus. A miscarriage is not done intentionally and so is not morally blameworthy. An induced abortion is immoral. Abortion is never considered as true therapy. Moralists add one more distinction: a) *Direct abortion*: One which is intended, even if its purpose is considered "therapeutic." The directly intended killing is always immoral. b) *Indirect abortion*: An abortion which is not directly intended, even though it may be foreseen as the result or side-effect of some other legitimate procedure. Under some circumstances this may not be immoral.

**Amniocentesis**: Puncturing of the amnion by passing a needle through the abdominal wall and the wall of the uterus, in order to withdraw a sample of the amniotic fluid.

**Amnion**: Part of the fetal organs. It is a fluid filled sac which surrounds and protects the fetus. It is often referred to as the "bag of waters."

**Amniotic Fluid**: An almost colorless fluid contained in the amniotic sac (the amnion) and surrounding the fetus.

**Amniotic Sac**: See *Amnion*.

**Anatomy**: The branch of science which treats of the structure of the body and the relationship of its parts.

353

**Antibody:** A substance which reacts to overcome the toxic effects of antigens. Some antibodies exist naturally in blood serum; others are produced when an antigen is introduced.

**Antigen:** A substance produced by the body in order to bring about the production of antibodies.

**Artificial Insemination:** The injection of semen into the vagina or uterus by means of a syringe rather than by sexual intercourse.

**Basal Temperature:** The body temperature at a standard low level of activity. It is the temperature taken immediately upon waking and before conducting any kind of activity at all.

**Bilirubin:** A reddish pigment, found in bile, in feces and in urine (when there is jaundice).

**Biologist:** A scientist who deals with living beings and their life forms in general.

**Biomedical Ethics:** That part of ethics or moral theology which deals with life issues in the context of the science of medicine.

**Biomedicine:** Clinical medicine which deals with relationships between body chemistry and body function.

**CAT Scan:** Computer Assisted Tomography. A much more sophisticated use of X-ray in which a moving camera, aided by computer, is able to produce a series of pictures in order to scan a whole area of the body, such as the brain.

**Central Nervous System:** The part of the nervous system which is composed of the brain and the spinal cord.

**Cervix:** The Latin word for neck. It is used in the context of this book to refer to the cervix or narrow lower end of the uterus.

**Chorionic Gonadotropic Hormone:** A substance produced by the chorion and found in the urine of pregnant women.

**Chorion:** The outermost fetal membrane. The part of it having villi, in which are blood vessels, forms the fetal portion of the placenta.

**Chorionic Villi:** Minute projections (hairlike or worm like structures) in which are blood vessels. The villi embed in the uterine wall and enable nourishment and waste to pass back and forth between mother and child.

**Chorionic Villus Sampling:** See *CVS*.

**Chromosome:** Small bodies in the nucleus of living cells. They carry the genes. In a human being, each cell has 46 chromosomes. Of these,

23 come from the sperm of the father and 23 from the egg of the mother.

**Clomid**: A drug (Clomiphene Citrate) used to induce ovulation. It acts as a receptor barrier, preventing the hormonal messages which indicate rises in estrogen and progesterone.

**Clone**: An individual obtained by asexual reproduction from a single original individual.

**Computer Assisted Tomography**: See *CAT SCAN*.

**Consent, informed**: Consent which is given and obtained on the basis of full and appropriate communication of information.

**Cryopreservation**: The preservation of living things by the reduction of body temperature to freezing.

**CVS**: Chorionic Villus Sampling. A surgical procedure in which some villi from the chorion of a fetus are removed, usually in order to conduct genetic tests in order to diagnose certain abnormalities.

**Cytologist**: One who studies that part of biology which deals with cells.

**Diagnosis**: The art of finding out the nature of disease in a patient.

**Down's Syndrome**: Also called Trisomy 21 or Mongolism. A hereditary disorder caused by an extra chromosome. It results in certain distinctive physical features and varying degrees of mental retardation.

**Duct System**: A system of tubes or channels within the body, such as the portion of the sexual anatomy in either male or female which conduct the sperm or egg to appropriate places.

**Dyspareunia**: Painful sexual intercourse.

**Egg**: The ovum; the female germ cell. Its nucleus carries the 23 chromosomes which come from the mother. It is fertilized by sperm. The egg is the largest single cell in a human body.

**Electroencephalogram**: Also referred to as EEG. A record produced by an instrument for measuring and recording electrical activity of the brain.

**Embryo**: The unborn child from the time of fertilization until the end of the eighth week of pregnancy.

**Embryology**: The study of the embryo and its development.

**Endocrine Glands**: Glands which secrete hormones directly into the blood stream. Ovaries and testes, although they produce eggs and sperm, are also endocrine glands and produce various hormones.

**Endocrinology**: Study of endocrine glands and their functions.

**Endometrium**: The blood-rich inner lining of the uterus. It is this tissue which breaks down and is expelled in the menstrual flow each month. It is also in this tissue that the embryo implants itself.

**Endometriosis**: The presence of endometrial tissue in places other than the inner wall of the uterus. It may appear on ovaries, in the fallopian tubes or in various other places. This condition is frequently a factor in cases of infertility.

**Erythroblast**: An immature red blood cell.

**Erythroblastosis fetalis**: A form of anemia in the fetus, due to adverse reaction to antibodies in the blood of the mother. (This is dealt with in detail in the text.)

**Erythrocyte**: A mature red blood cell. The erythrocyte is disk shaped; it carries oxygen throughout the body and is responsible for the color of blood.

**Estrogen**: One of the hormones responsible for the bodily changes which take place during a woman's monthly cycle. It is produced both naturally and synthetically.

**ET**: Embryo transfer. The term is generally used to refer to the transfer of an embryo into a woman's body after fertilization has taken place in a petri dish.

**Eugenism**: A theory dealing with genetic improvement of the human race.

**Euthanasia**: Mercy killing. The direct destruction of a human life.

**Fallopian Tubes**: The tube which transports the egg from the ovary into the uterus. It is usually in the upper third of the tube that conception takes place.

**Fetoscopy**: A procedure in which a needle containing a light and a fiberoptic lens is inserted into the amnion in order to view the fetus.

**Fetus**: The developing child in the uterus from the end of the eighth week of pregnancy until the time of birth.

**Fimbria**: Literally, fringe. The fringelike upper end of the fallopian tube. Its movement draws the ripe ovum into the end of the tube so that it can be passed on into the uterus.

**Fistula**: A narrow passage or opening produced by disease or injury.

**Follicle**: A small cavity or sac. In the context of this book the word is used to refer to the small sacs in which the egg develops on the surface of the ovary.

356

**Follicle Stimulating Hormone:** A hormone produced by the pituitary gland which regulates development of the ovarian follicles in the female and stimulates sperm production in the male.

**FSH:** See *Follicle Stimulating Hormone*.

**Gamete:** A reproductive cell (the egg in the female and sperm in the male).

**Gene:** The physical unit of heredity. Genes are attached to specific places on particular chromosomes.

**Genetics:** The study of the factors of heredity.

**Gestational:** Pertaining to gestation, which is the process from conception to birth.

**GIFT:** Gamete Intrafallopian Transfer. A process used to assist in certain problems with fertility. Gametes (egg and sperm) are placed in the upper end of the fallopian tube, where conception can take place *in vivo*.

**Gonadotropic:** Referring to substances which affect the activity of the ovary or testicles.

**HCG:** Human Chorionic Gonadotropic Hormone. This is a hormone produced in the placenta and acts to signal the body of the woman of its need to sustain pregnancy.

**Hormone:** A chemical substance produced by glands and having effects on other organs or functions.

**Hypothalamus:** A portion of the brain.

**Hysterotomy:** The cutting of an opening into the uterus. This is part of the procedure performed in a Caesarian Section. It is also the word used now to describe the process of cutting into the womb in order to abort children.

**Implantation:** The embedding of the embryo into the endometrium.

**Infertility:** The incapacity to conceive or bear children. The causes vary widely and may be traced to either or both partners.

**Intrafallopian Transfer:** A surgical procedure in which egg or sperm are placed into the fallopian tube as an aid in cases of infertility.

**Invasive:** Referring to techniques of diagnosis or treatment which involve some sort of physical entrance into the body or its organs.

**In vitro:** Literally it means "in glass." *In vitro* fertilization refers to a process in which an egg is fertilized by sperm in a petri dish rather than in the body of the mother.

**In vivo**: Literally it means "inside a living being." *In vivo* fertilization refers to the fertilization of an egg by sperm within the body of a woman.

**IVF**: An abbreviation for "*in vitro* fertilization." See *in vitro*.

**Laparoscopy**: A process of introducing a light and lens through an incision in the abdomen in order to view internal organs.

**LH**: See *Luteinizing Hormone*.

**LTOT**: Lower Tubal Ovarian Transfer. A surgical procedure in which the ovum is moved into the lower part of the fallopian tube for the purpose of fertilization. It is done in cases where blockage of the tube prevents movement of the egg.

**Lung Maturity**: The stage of fetal lung development at which it becomes possible for the fetus to breath air. This happens at about the twenty-fourth week of pregnancy and is the earliest point at which a fetus is viable.

**Luteinizing Hormone**: A hormone produced by the pituitary gland. In the female it regulates the development of the corpus luteum. In the male it stimulates the production of testosterone. It is also referred to as LH or ICSH (Interstitial Cell Stimulating Hormone).

**Magnetic Resonance Imaging (MRI)**: A technique which uses radio waves and a magnetic field to produce images. Unlike X-ray, it ignores hard tissue such as bone, and forms very useful images of soft tissue.

**Menstruation**: The discharging of blood and tissue from the uterus during a woman's monthly cycle.

**Metrodin**: A drug used to stimulate the production of eggs in the ovary. It contains both FSH and LH.

**Miscarriage**: A spontaneous, accidental, non-induced abortion.

**Mongolism**: See *Down's Syndrome*:

**MRI**: See *Magnetic Resonance Imaging*.

**Non-invasive**: Referring to techniques of diagnosis or therapy which do not involve physical entrance into the body or its organs.

**Ovarian Stimulation**: The use of drugs to cause the ovaries to produce eggs.

**Ovary**: One of a pair of sex glands in the female. Contains the follicle from which the eggs mature. Also responsible for production of various hormones.

**Ovulation**: The process by which the woman's eggs mature and are released. Each month one egg comes to maturity in one of the ovaries.

358

**Ovum**: See *Egg*.

**Parthenogenesis**: Literally, "virgin birth." Development of an organism from an unfertilized egg.

**Pelvic Inflammatory Disease (PID)**: A generic term referring to various types of infection in the pelvic area. These infections frequently begin with diseases related to sexual activity and can become serious enough to cause permanent damage or even death.

**Pergonal**: A combination of synthetic FSH and synthetic LH used to stimulate production of eggs in the ovary.

**Petri Dish**: A shallow covered dish in which cell cultures are grown. Also used for fertilizing eggs in IVF.

**Photosynthesis**: The process by which green plants are able to use water, carbon dioxide, minerals and light to produce food.

**Physiology**: The science which examines the functions of bodily organs.

**PID**: See *Pelvic Inflammatory Disease*.

**Placenta**: The fetal organ by which the fetus is attached to the wall of the uterus. The umbilical cord runs from the placenta to the fetus and through its blood vessels nourishment and waste are exchanged with the mother.

**Placenta Previa**: A condition in which the placenta is situated in the uterus in such a way as to either completely or partially block the opening. It gives rise to serious bleeding during delivery.

**Premature infant**: A child born before the thirty-seventh week of pregnancy.

**Progesterone**: A hormone which prepares the uterus for the fertilized ovum and maintains pregnancy.

**Prostaglandin**: A substance which affects the nervous system, circulatory system and female reproductive organs. High concentrations of Prosteglandin are found in normal human semen.

**Rh factor**: An antigen carried on the surface of blood cells. Blood is classified as Rh-positive or Rh-negative, depending on whether this antigen is present or not. The "Rh" is an abbreviation for Rhesus (a type of monkey in which this factor was first discovered).

**Rhesus incompatibility**: The cause of erythroblastosis fetalis.

**Selective Reduction**: A form of abortion. The random killing of fetuses when there are deemed to be too many in a multiple pregnancy.

**Sickle Cell Anemia:** A disease in which red blood cells are distorted in shape, being sickle-shaped rather than disk-shaped. It is most commonly found in those of African origin.

**Silastic Sheath:** A type of condom. It is used for the gathering of sperm for analysis. It is perforated and allows the first of portion of the ejaculation to enter the vagina but then seals itself to maintain the rest of the semen.

**Sonography:** A technique for using ultrasound waves (beyond the range of human hearing) to penetrate tissue in order to produce a televised image of internal organs.

**Sperm:** The male reproductive cell. Hundreds of millions of sperm are contained in ejaculated semen.

**Suction Pump:** A pump used to suck the torn parts of a fetus from the uterus in the process of abortion.

**Surfactant:** A substance on the alveoli (air sacs of the lung). Its presence in the amniotic fluid is a sign of lung maturity in the fetus. This is important as an indication of viability.

**Surrogate Motherhood:** The impregnation of a woman with a man's sperm, with the understanding (arranged by contract) that the child will be given to the sperm donor and his wife and will be legally their child. Legal status of such an arrangement is currently unclear.

**Sympto-thermal Method:** A method for determining the time of ovulation in the woman's monthly cycle. It examines the symptoms indicated in body temperature and cervical mucus.

**Tay-Sachs Disease:** A severe hereditary disorder leading to death by the age of three or four. It is almost always found in those of Eastern European Jewish origin.

**Term:** The time of delivery of a baby.

**Testis:** One of a pair of sex glands in the male. They produce sperm and hormones.

**Testosterone:** The male sex hormone produced by the testes and responsible for the development of masculine characteristics.

**Thalassemia:** A form of anemia resulting from hereditary defects. It is found in those of Mediterranean or Oriental origin and has varying degrees of seriousness.

**Therapy:** The process of bringing about a cure or the proper management of a disease.

**Trimester**:  A period of three months.  One of the three three-month segments which make up the nine months of pregnancy.

**Trisomy 21**:  See *Down's Syndrome*.

**Trisomy**:  The presence of an extra chromosome in a pair.  In a human being this would mean the presence of 47 instead of 46 chromosomes.  Usually results in some form of abnormality.  For example, Trisomy 21 would mean an extra chromosome in the twenty-first pair, which would result in Down's Syndrome.

**Twin Fission**:  The division of a single fertilized egg into twins.

**Ultrasound**:  Sound waves beyond the range of human hearing.  They are used in sonography.

**Uterus**:  The womb.  A pear-shaped, muscular organ.  The site of pregnancy where the fertilized ovum implants and grows until birth.

**Utilitarianism**:  A system of thought which judges the value of things and persons on the basis of their usefulness and not because of their own intrinsic value.

**Varicocele**:  A varicose vein on the spermatic cords of the scrotum.  It can interfere with male fertility.

**Varicose Veins**:  Veins which are abnormally swollen or enlarged.

**Viability**:  The state of the fetus when it is able to live outside the uterus.

**Villi**:  Plural of "villus."  Hairlike appendages of mucus membrane containing a system of vessels for blood or lymph. They are found, for example, on the inner surface of the intestines or on the outer surface of the chorion.

**X-Ray**:  Electromagnetic radiation capable of passing through solids, such as the human body, and producing an image on a photographic plate.

**ZIFT**:  Zygote Intrafollopian Transfer.  A form of *in vitro* fertilization in which eggs are fertilized in a petri dish and, in the Zygote stage, are then transferred into the fallopian tube.

**Zygote**:  The fertilized egg, before it begins to divide into further cells.

# BIBLIOGRAPHY

# BIBLIOGRAPHY

Ashley, Benedict M., and O'Rourke, Kevin, *Health Care Ethics*, Catholic Hospital Association, St. Louis, Missouri, 1982.

Berkow, Robert, *ed., The Merck Manual, Fifteenth Edition*, Merck, Sharp and Dohme Research Laboratories, Rahway, New Jersey, 1987.

Carroll, Lewis, *Alice in Wonderland*, 1865.

Carroll, Lewis, *Through the Looking-Glass*, 1872.

Cuomo, Mario M., "Religious Belief and Public Morality: A Catholic Governor's Perspective," a paper prepared for delivery to the Department of Theology at the University of Notre Dame, September 13, 1984.

Hamilton, Edith, *Mythology*, Mentor Books, New York, 1963.

Horan, Dennis J., and Balch, Burke J., "Infant Doe and Baby Jane Doe: Medical Treatment of the Handicapped Newborn," in *Linacre Quarterly*, Vol. 52, 1985, pp. 45-76.

Huff, Barbara B., *ed., 1989 Physicians' Desk Reference*, Medical Economics Company, Oradell, New Jersey, 1989 (43rd edition).

Johnstone, Brian V., "The Sanctity of Life, the Quality of Life and the New 'Baby Doe' law," in *Linacre Quarterly*, Vol, 52, 1985, pp. 258-270.

Lejeune, Jerome, Testimony in the Knoxville "frozen embryos" case of 1989, recorded by Peggy M. Giles, Knoxville Court Reporting.

Lewis, C.S., *The Weight of Glory*, Wm. B. Erdmans Publishing Co., Grand Rapids, Michigan, 1966.

McCarthy, Donald G., *ed., Reproductive Technologies, Marriage and the Church*, Pope John XXIII Research Center, Braintree, Massachusetts, 1988.

Menning, Barbara Eck, *Infertility: A Guide for the Childless Couple*, Prentice Hall Press, New York, 1977, 1988.

O'Donnell, Thomas J., *Medicine and Christian Morality*, Alba House, New York, 1976.

Rini, Suzanne M., *Beyond Abortion: A Chronicle of Fetal Experimentation*, Magnificat Press, Avon-by-the-Sea, New Jersey, 1988.

Sacred Congregation for the Doctrine of the Faith, *Declaration on Procured Abortion (Quaestio de abortu)*, November 18, 1974. English text may be found in *Vatican Council II: More Postconciliar Documents*, Austin Flannery, *ed.*, Liturgical Press, Collegeville, MN. pp. 441-453.

Sagan, Carl, and Druyan, Ann, "Is it possible to be Pro-Life and Pro-Choice?" in *Parade Magazine*, April 22, 1990, 4-8.

Stoppard, Doctor Miriam, *Everywoman's Medical Handbook*, Ballantine Books, New York, 1989.

Supreme Court, Opinions given in the case of Webster v. Reproductive Health Services, in *Origins, CNS Documentary Service*, July 13, 1989, Vol. 19: No. 9, pp. 129-151.

Supreme Court, *Doe v. Bolton*, October 11, 1970, arguments in No. 70-40, official transcript acquired from Federal Document Retrieval, 810 First street N.E. Suite 600, Washington, D.C.

Supreme Court, *Doe v. Bolton*, December 13, 1971, arguments in No. 70-40, official transcript acquired from Federal Document Retrieval, 810 First street N.E. Suite 600, Washington, D.C.

Supreme Court, *Roe v. Wade*, December 13, 1971, arguments in No. 70-18, official transcript acquired from Federal Document Retrieval, 810 First street N.E. Suite 600, Washington, D.C.

Supreme Court, *Roe v. Wade*, October 11, 1972, arguments in No. 70-18, official transcript acquired from Federal Document Retrieval, 810 First street N.E. Suite 600, Washington, D.C.

Wallace, Marilyn, and Hilgers, Thomas, *eds., The Gift of Life: The Proceedings of a National Conference on the Vatican Instruction on Reproductive Ethics and Technology*, Pope Paul VI Institute Press, Omaha, Nebraska, 1990.

Varii, *The New York Times*, articles and authors cited where quoted.

Weinstein, Kate, *Living with Endometriosis*, Addison-Wesley Publishing Company, New York, 1987.

Willke, Doctor and Mrs. J.C., *Abortion: Questions and Answers*, Hays Publishing Company, Inc., Cincinnati, Ohio, 1985.

Wlazelek, Ann, and Slaten, Rosa, Series of articles on Fertility in *The Allentown Morning Call*, Allentown, Pennsylvania, July 30, 1989 (pp. A1, B20-21); July 31, 1989 (pp. D1-2, D8); August 1, 1989 (pp. D1, D6).

INDEX

# INDEX

371

382